AIDS AND LOCAL GOVERNMENT IN SOUTH AFRICA

EXAMINING THE IMPACT OF AN EPIDEMIC ON WARD COUNCILLORS

BY KONDWANI CHIRAMBO AND JUSTIN STEYN

WITH ADDITIONAL RESEARCH BY CHRISTELE DIWOUTA AND NJINGA KANKINZA

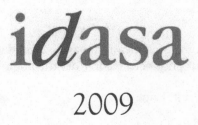

2009

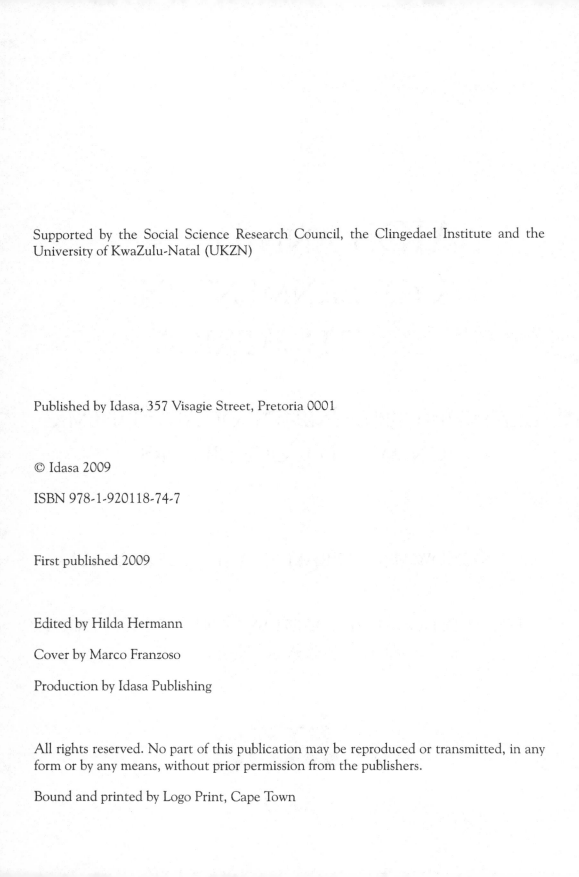

Supported by the Social Science Research Council, the Clingedael Institute and the University of KwaZulu-Natal (UKZN)

Published by Idasa, 357 Visagie Street, Pretoria 0001

ISBN 978-1-920118-74-7

First published 2009

Edited by Hilda Hermann

Cover by Marco Franzoso

Production by Idasa Publishing

Bound and printed by Logo Print, Cape Town

ACKNOWLEDGEMENTS

This work has been made possible through the support of the Netherlands Institute for International Relations (CLINGEDAEL), the Social Sciences Research Council and the University of KwaZulu-Natal (UKZN). I take this opportunity to sincerely commend them for their support.

The project was conceived and researched by Idasa as a contribution to the AIDS, Security and Conflict Initiative (ASCI). The execution of this research was aided by Citizen Surveys, which administered the bulk of the questionnaires prepared by Idasa to enable wider coverage in a relatively short period. AfriGIS developed the maps and generated the statistical summations for Idasa.

Our gratitude is also extended to Hermien Kotze, who contributed to the review of questionnaires and coordinated the fieldwork involving Idasa-Governance and AIDS Programme (GAP) researchers and Citizen Surveys. Finally, I wish to thank Marietjie Myburg and Vailet Mukotsanjera, our two regional coordinators, for communication and AIDS budgets respectively; and for their contributions at various stages of the project. Jennifer Dreyer, as always, supported the process with her diligent administrative work.

Kondwani Chirambo
Programme Manager

AUTHORS AND RESEARCHERS

Kondwani Chirambo is director of Idasa-GAP. Chirambo pioneered research on the impact of HIV/AIDS on the electoral process in Africa in 2003, and has subsequently led several regional research projects covering the political process. His recent publications include: *Democratisation in the Age of HIV/AIDS: Understanding the political implications* (2006) and *The Political Cost of AIDS in Africa* (2008), both published by Idasa. Chirambo is a Doctoral Candidate in Communication Science with the University of South Africa (UNISA).

Justin Steyn is a researcher with Idasa-GAP. He is PhD scholar at the University of the Witwatersrand, Johannesburg. His focus has been on political philosophy and its effect on free agency in active social engagement.

Christele Diwouta is a researcher with Idasa-GAP. She holds an LLM in Human Rights and Democratisation from the University of Pretoria; a Maitrise in Business Law from the University of Dschang, Cameroon, and an LLB from the University of Buea, Cameroon. Christele worked as research assistant with the Centre for the Study of AIDS and has observed elections in Madagascar and Nigeria organised with the Electoral Institute of Southern Africa (EISA) and Idasa respectively. She has contributed to publications facilitated by Idasa on HIV/AIDS and child labour.

Njinga Kankinza holds an Honours in Psychology from the University of Pretoria. She works as an intern at Idasa-GAP.

EXECUTIVE SUMMARY

This study seeks to understand "how AIDS epidemics can contribute to state fragility" (Cluster C of the AIDS, Security and Conflict Initiative [ASCI].) An exploratory project, the study does not aim to measure fragility but to identify trends that may introduce it. A fragile state is generally defined as one characterised by weak governance, poor service delivery and ineffective policies. Indicators of state fragility encapsulate political, economic, humanitarian and social dimensions (Hannan & Besada: 2007; Rice & Patrick: 2008). The study sampled 12 local municipalities in the Western Cape, Northern Cape, Free State and KwaZulu-Natal, with the aim of comprehending the impact of HIV/AIDS on ward councillors, and the epidemic's potential to affect accountability, effective government and legitimacy. In this context, the study will unpack seven central themes relating to the political domain of governance:

- The implications of the depletion of leadership through mortality and the consequent loss of institutional memory in local government.
- The shifting configuration of power in local government due to by-elections and its implications for democratic accountability.
- The economic costs of replacing deceased councillors and sustainability of electoral models.
- The impact of stigma and discrimination, and functionality of leadership, at local level.
- Community perceptions of HIV-positive councillors and service delivery.
- The impact of voter mortality on political legitimacy.
- The local government response to HIV/AIDS (and its potential to minimise leadership and staff attrition).

Within these seven points, this study focuses primarily on 3 895 directly elected ward councillors (out of 8 951 councillors nationwide). At the time of this research, 5 056 councillors were appointed through the proportional representation (PR) system. The focus on councillors is partly motivated by the important role they are expected to play in development within a country currently challenged to uplift the welfare of millions of historically disadvantaged people amidst service delivery backlogs. Afrobarometer studies indicate that South Africans pass judgment on the efficacy of local government mainly based on the perceived performances of their councillors, whom they expect to act as agents of change and development (Bratton & Sibanyoni: 2006). A disruption of this delicate linkage between governor and governed in highly volatile environments could contribute to heightened perceptions of poor governance. Increased mortality and morbidity on a broad scale may cripple local authorities already grappling with the effects of skills shortages.

The study assumes that attrition of skills due to AIDS, loss of professionals to other sectors of the economy and increasing demands of service delivery may conspire to undermine local authorities, as some related studies suggest (Whiteside & Sunter: 2000: Isandla: 2007). AIDS infects 5,4 million South Africans, of whom 18% are economically active (Dorrington, et al.: 2006).

METHODS

The methods used for this study include interviews with elected officials in local government, the Independent Electoral Commission (IEC) of South Africa, HIV/AIDS managers in local government, municipal managers and Integrated Development Plan (IDP) managers. This group served to inform the study on matters relating to mortality among councillors, the frequency and costs of by-elections held to replace deceased councillors, the impact of HIV/AIDS on the administrative system and its ability to support the political system, and, finally, the institutional arrangements available to sustain the AIDS sick. Statistical analysis of electoral data and HIV/AIDS data provided a basis for drawing inferences on the potential AIDS deaths among the elected representatives and registered voters who form part of their communities. Focus group discussions with community members assisted us to understand levels of expectation in terms of service delivery, and the impact of stigma and discrimination on the work of councillors who may be infected by HIV. Extensive literature reviews of AIDS journals, publications on state fragility, local government reports and Afrobarometer studies on local government were also undertaken.

BACKGROUND

The practical experience of democratic local government in South Africa is barely eight years old. While South Africa's 1996 Constitution defined how society would be administered by a three-tier system of government – national, provincial and local – it was not until 2000 that the current structure of local government began to be modelled and operationalised. In terms of the 1996 Constitution, four interactive systems would define municipal government: the institutional system, the political system, the administrative system and the financial system.

The institutional system defines and divides local government into three categories of municipal authority: category A municipalities, which are larger industrialised zones often referred to as metros; category B municipalities, which are also referred to as local councils; and category C municipalities, which are district municipal authorities comprising a variable number of category B structures. A total of 283 municipalities were established after the first local government election in 2000 under the new structures and laws.[1] The Municipal Structures Act of 1998 and the Municipal Systems Act of 2000 defined the political structure and the function of local government authorities respectively. Governance, as stipulated in the Acts, would be cooperative, or what we may describe as integrated and sectorally interdisciplinary. Cooperation in delivering on the developmental mandate would be functional across tiers and across departmental functions, as mandated in Chapter Three of the Constitution.

As structural entities, local councils would be demand-driven by the communities' need for services. This need would be addressed by elected representatives comprising the political system, who form the council structure and ward committees. Locally elected representatives would facilitate the participation of the community in IDPs and the Local Economic Development (LED) programmes, an approach framed as a developmental model by the South African government. These programmes would incorporate community needs into the planning processes (Municipal Systems Act 2000: Chapter 4). The implementation of programmes, and the allocation and monitoring of resources, would be achieved through the administrative and financial systems respectively.[2]

State-led initiatives had, as early as 2002, recognised the inherent weaknesses and challenges faced by the new local government structure in South Africa. Not only had the demand for equitable services increased with the achievement of a democratic dispensation, but also the need for a sound skills base to deliver on the expectations of millions was apparent. Failure to retain and develop scarce skills was a key concern of the government's 'Project Consolidate'. In its review of 2004, 'Project Consolidate' revealed that municipalities were not institutionally prepared to perform their traditional local government functions of providing water and sanitation services, and other related tasks. What is noticeable from the 2004–2006 'Project Consolidate' document is the omission of HIV/AIDS as a significant factor that might undermine the sustainability of local governance. The epidemic was not defined as a core integrated part of municipal business (DPLG: 2007). This was despite reports about the potential for HIV/AIDS to undermine the effectiveness of governance through absenteeism and loss of institutional memory (Whiteside and Sunter: 2001).

Over time, response frameworks crafted by the Department of Provincial and Local Government (DPLG) and the South African Local Government Association (SALGA) provided a basis for defining a more strategic role for councillors, professional staff and local authorities in general in relation to HIV/AIDS in South Africa. The notion of mainstreaming is factored into managerial interventions that seek to mitigate impact on communities and provide political leadership (DPLG: 2007; SALGA: 2008). The SALGA strategy of 2008 emphasises the use of political structures, such as ward committees supported by ward councillors to undertake situational analysis, identify service gaps and work out coordinated responses with Non-Governmental Organisations (NGOs). It notes that some councils have used community-based forums in the absence of ward committees to create multisectoral AIDS teams at local level. The document notably recognises the need for training and further knowledge building to make these interventions effective. Overall, there is recognition that a local response to HIV/AIDS is work-in-progress that demands not only strong leadership, but also cross-sectoral partnerships (SALGA: 2008:24). There is no critical analysis in the document of the potential impact of HIV/AIDS and its ramifications for local capacity to effectively utilise these blueprints.

FINDINGS

THE IMPLICATIONS OF THE DEPLETION OF LEADERSHIP THROUGH MORTALITY AND THE CONSEQUENT LOSS OF INSTITUTIONAL MEMORY IN LOCAL GOVERNMENT

This study is fore-grounded by a discussion suggesting that HIV/AIDS could reduce the range of available skills and institutional memory, given South Africa's current skills deficit. With its relatively short history of running democratic local government, South Africa is likely to face a severe challenge if it is unable to retain or sustain skilled and experienced personnel in its political, administrative and financial systems.

The political system – essentially the decision-making arm of local government – is complimented by the administrative system, which is the implementing wing of this tier of government. Based on an extensive literature review, which includes public opinion data from Afrobarometer and news reports, we make the case that matters of local governance in South Africa are extremely volatile due to high expectations among previously disadvantaged populations who have, in the recent past, resorted to violent means to register their displeasure at the performance of councillors and government. We suggest that, should AIDS or other causes generate repeated vacancies in the political system of local government, the disruptions to the relationship between councillors and their communities may contribute to a state of polarisation between the governors and governed, and further accentuate the perception of non-delivery that seems to have gained momentum over the last five years. The means by which we track mortality among the 3 895 ward councillors nationwide is through the occurrence and recurrence of by-elections. By identifying the cause of by-elections, assessing the ages of the deceased, and observing trends, we are able to draw inferences on whether the mortality patterns correspond to those generally associated with HIV/AIDS.

In this context, the study found that 589 by-elections were held between 28 February 2001 and December 2007 throughout South Africa. Of these, 285 were caused by deaths of ward councillors. Some 241 by-elections were due to councillors resigning their positions, 44 were sacked, five expelled and two imprisoned, resulting in further by-elections during the same period. Death accounts for 48,7% of all vacancies compared to resignation at 40,9%, termination of councillor membership by party at 7,5%, dissolution of council by Members of Executive Committees (MECs) 2,0%, expulsions 0,8%, and imprisonment 0,1%. The data shows that male deaths totalled 217. In 2001, male councillors in the 25–29 and 35–39 age groups accounted for 21% of all the deaths among this gender, while the 60–64 age cohort accounted for only 3,4%. The largest number of councillors to die came from the 45–49 age group, which accounted for 23% of the deaths. There is no distinct pattern when female and male deaths are compared. The female mortality patterns are characterised by regular fluctuations. While there are no corresponding patterns in general between the two data sets, we have noted that there is a concentration of deaths in both sexes in the economically active population aged 29–42. The most critical observation from this study is that the life expectancy among councillors appears to be 51 years. To support the assertion that AIDS may be the main explanation, reference is made to expert demographers who indicate that life expectancy in South Africa has reduced from 64 to 51 years due to AIDS (Dorrington, et al.: 2006). In an earlier report, Dorrington, et al. (2004) also indicated that 70% of all deaths in 2004 in the age group 15–49 years were due to AIDS. The figure declined to 45% when all adults (aged 15+) were factored in. Taking this AIDS ratio as a constant for the 2001–2007 period, the conclusion is inferred that 70% of local councillors in the 22–49 age cohort died of AIDS. This reasoning is qualified by the following assumptions:

- Councillors are universally representative of all South Africans.
- Councillor gender is of a representative parity.
- A constant AIDS death ratio applies to all South Africa for the period 2001–2007.
- The consistent distribution of HIV/AIDS prevails across the entire country.

In absolute terms, the 22–49 years olds who died during this period numbered 233. It means that, of these, 163 will have died of AIDS.

Dorrington, et al. (2006) suggest further that, without a treatment programme, the decline in life expectancy will be almost 19 years by 2015, with the average life expectancy falling to 48 years. With an Anti-retroviral Therapy (ART) programme, average life expectancy would be 50 years. Personal accounts from ward councillors, in the 112 interviews conducted, suggest that they are aware of AIDS-related deaths among their ranks, and among close friends and family more generally. Of the respondents, 59,4% said they had lost a family member, relation or friend to AIDS. 16,8% said they knew a fellow councillor/s that had died of the disease. One way AIDS will impact on governance is by robbing communities of their preferred representatives, which may paralyse decision making on their set priorities unless effective substitutes are appointed. The study does, however, find that South Africa's local government system provides for administrative mechanisms to deal with communities in the period when there is no representative (either due to death, resignation or expulsion). These include the speaker of council taking care of the matters of the community; a temporary councillor being appointed to fill the seat left by the deceased while a by-election is organised; or a ward coordinator or liaison officer being assigned to engage with the community he or she represents. In this sense, the conclusion is drawn that the loss of a representative will not necessarily lead to ineffectiveness, as long as the mechanisms are consistently applied in all wards where vacancies occur.

However, there are some concerns still to be raised regarding the efficacy of these measures in terms of service delivery. The Auditor-General's 2006/2007 report reveals the inability of municipalities to meet the needs of their communities. According to the report, some 60% of municipalities cannot reconcile expenditure with receipts. The Auditor-General also draws a link between poor financial and administrative capacity and the current political instability in the country over lack of service delivery (*Mail & Guardian* 20/06/08). Given this revelation, doubts are raised as to whether substitute councillors or liaison officers will be able to enable effective government, particularly since they have to rely on the administrative and financial systems that are adjudged by professional auditors as largely incapable of efficient delivery. In addition, will the communities consider a Proportional Representation (PR) councillor, a liaison officer or a ward coordinator a legitimate substitute for a directly elected ward councillor?

THE SHIFTING CONFIGURATION OF POWER IN LOCAL GOVERNMENT DUE TO BY-ELECTIONS AND ITS IMPLICATIONS FOR DEMOCRATIC ACCOUNTABILITY

In the analyses of patterns emerging from by-election outcomes, some shifts in representation in the local authority structures are noted. From the 589 by-elections held between 2001 and 2007, the major beneficiary has been the ruling African National Congress (ANC). During the six years, the ANC won a total of 47 by-elections, but also surrendered 16, leaving its net gain at 31. The most affected, each recording negative growth, have been the Inkatha Freedom Party (IFP), the United Democratic Movement (UDM), the Democratic Alliance (DA) and the New National Party (NNP), which was absorbed into the ANC subsequent to the 2004 national elections. The information raises the possibility of a weakened opposition in the local government sector. Given the myriad issues associated with local government in South Africa, it may be logical to assume that the presence of a robust, energetic opposition is likely to raise the level of answerability and accountability as the party in power will constantly try to prove its worth through improved service delivery. There are three ways in which AIDS is likely to affect accountability:

- The opposition will be further weakened as its numbers dwindle in council, affecting its effectiveness as a counterweight to the ruling party.
- Secondly, the dominant party may become less responsive to community needs due to low threat perception from an opposition in decline (otherwise reactive, rather than proactive, to the needs of communities).
- Conversely, a dominant party may be effective, wary of surrendering territory to the opposition in the foreseeable future.

THE ECONOMIC COSTS OF REPLACING DECEASED COUNCILLORS AND SUSTAINABILITY OF ELECTORAL MODELS

Replacing deceased leaders has four implications:

- The Mixed Member Proportional (MMP) system, an electoral model partly based on majoritarian principles, may be unsustainable due to rising economic costs.
- Small political parties that are not represented in parliament will not be able to afford to compete in every by-election (parliamentary parties in South Africa receive state funding proportionate to the number of seats won in the last general election).
- Frequent by-elections may impact on the productivity of local communities, who would lose opportunities to contribute to the economy more directly by participating in numerous polls.
- By-elections may impact on the legitimacy of the winner as too few people turn up at each poll to cast ballots.

The cost of by-elections is borne by the IEC, the local authorities and the political party. According to Michael Hendrickse, a senior officer at the IEC, a ward by-election costs on average R25 000 (US$3 333).[3] Based on this figure, South Africa has spent at least R14,7 million (US$1,9 million) on hosting by-elections between 2001 and 2007. At least half of that amount, R7,1 million (US$946 667), was spent on 285 wards where councillors died of undisclosed causes, compared to R6 million (US$800 000) to fill vacancies caused by resignations, R1 million (US$133 333) due to termination of services of councillors and R300 000 (US$40 000) for the dissolution of council. We note that deaths among councillors generate more costs to the MMP system than other causes. Investigations confirm that, while the costs of by-elections appear to be high, the IEC has enough funding to finance them at this point in time (Interview: Hendrickse). Municipalities, which are also required to support the process, however, indicate that the task of holding by-elections tends to be arduous, particularly given their other capacity deficits. While the IEC may at this stage not be strained financially by elections, we need to consider opportunity costs that are beyond the scope of this study – for example, advertising, administrative expenses and fieldwork carried out by political parties during elections. Numerous by-elections will favour parliamentary parties that are awarded state funds based on their previous electoral performance.

Repeated elections do not bode well for the emergent political parties seeking to gain access to decision-making mechanisms. It needs to be stated further that, even among parliamentary parties, the resources are not distributed equally. Political party funding is determined through the Public Funding of Represented Political Parties Act (PFRPPA) of 1997. Its provisions state that political parties shall be allocated public funds in proportion to the number of seats they hold in the National Assembly and provincial legislatures in order to reinforce the idea of proportionality in representation (PFRPPA of 1997 5[2][a]). From the allocation, 90% is paid at the start of the financial year. The allocation is proportional to the number of seats each political party averages in the provincial and national legislature. The remaining 10% becomes a provincial allocation. The funds are divided according to the seats in each provincial legislature and each political party in each legislature takes an equal share of the allocation. Similarly, it could be assumed that some of the voters will be in gainful employment or involved in some form of economic activity. Their regular involvement in by-elections may reduce their contribution to the well-being of their communities in some respects.

THE IMPACT OF STIGMA AND DISCRIMINATION, AND FUNCTIONALITY OF LEADERSHIP, AT LOCAL LEVEL

We understand stigma and discrimination as impacting on effectiveness and accountability by causing the elected representative to withdraw from public functions or community forums, particularly when they exhibit visible signs of illness. We find that indeed, there is a general fear among ward councillors interviewed in this study that disclosure of one's HIV status could ruin political careers. This impression is widely shared among the ward councillors. On the one hand, councillors express a fear of rejection by the electorate, who may deem them unfit for office if they are known to be HIV-positive; on the other, they see a danger of political opposition presenting them as incapable of ruling. Throughout the study we found only one councillor who openly lives with HIV. She is the first elected representative, to our knowledge, known to openly live with HIV. Hers is an isolated case as many councillors did not disclose or speak freely on this issue, although some did offer opinions on how we should deal with people with HIV. The emerging data creates the impression that HIV/AIDS denialism permeates politics. Denial can contribute to the weakening of the relationship between the governors and the governed, as councillors may choose to be absent from duty due to illness or stigma. This would have the consequence of reducing their effectiveness in responding to the needs of their communities. Municipal managers cited no specific cases of councillor absenteeism, but respondents spoke generally that it does seem to affect all tiers of municipal structures. Concern must be expressed over the leadership role of councillors, given their expressed 'fears' of testing, disclosure, the knowledge gaps and apparent indication of poor political response to HIV/AIDS within their communities.

COMMUNITY PERCEPTIONS OF HIV-POSITIVE COUNCILLORS AND SERVICE DELIVERY

Despite previous studies, which show entrenched stigma and discrimination against People Living with HIV/AIDS (PLWHAs) in South Africa(see Jennings: 2002), the participants in this study would not be deterred by the possibility of electing a councillor who was living with HIV. The activist make-up of our focus groups may explain their accommodating views. A more detailed study employing public opinion surveys may be useful in unravelling the extent to which HIV-positive candidates will be acceptable to the wider public. As tends to be borne out in prior Idasa experience, the disadvantage of the focus group is that participants are likely to be swayed by dominant voices, particularly the older members of the group. These factors notwithstanding, this ASCI project finds that members of the community participating in eight of our focus-group discussions in the four provinces exhibit high expectations of service delivery from their councillors. Participants anticipated a radical change in their present circumstances, with demands for better housing, employment opportunities, medical care, social welfare and education characterising all the discussions. They were able to draw a linkage between having a job and the capacity to survive HIV/AIDS. While most said there had been improvements in anti-retroviral (ARV) access since 1994, they bemoaned the general lack of responsiveness from their local councillors in regard to their current situation. The dominant view suggests that councillors never meet their electioneering promises and are often too distant from matters relating to AIDS relief. This heightened level of expectation may be problematic for councillors who fail to deliver due to illness or withdrawal from public functions.

THE IMPACT OF VOTER MORTALITY ON POLITICAL LEGITIMACY

Voting age populations (VAP) and registered voters are significant to this study because these are the citizens who decide on who presides over public affairs. The premise here is that low participation is problematic for democracy. Voter mortality by itself will not impact on legitimacy, but there are a number of related factors that could:

- Voter mortality may decrease the voter pool, impacting on participation levels.
- AIDS illness could constrain registered voters from voting (this was noted in previous studies by Idasa – Strand & Chirambo: 2005; Chirambo: 2008).
- Care giving could constrain participation due to contending priorities of survival (ibid.).
- Stigma and discrimination may also have similar effects, as noted in rural KwaZulu-Natal (Strand & Chirambo: 2005).
- Repeated by-elections have a tendency to attract relatively fewer voters.

A changing demographic of voters is likely also to impact on the type of public choices that prevail. Political parties that rely on relatively younger voters (below age 49) for membership may, for example, find their electoral support bases whittled away by HIV/AIDS.

The second level of concern relates to participation: a proliferation of sick voters will reduce the number of people available to vote, possibly impacting on the legitimacy of the candidates. This may especially occur during by-elections, which will have lower participation than a general election. Some examples from this study indicate that nine out of the twelve municipalities that held by-elections between 2001 and 2003, none achieved 50% participation. In effect, seven municipalities failed to reach 38% turnout in the by-elections held during the 2001–2003 period.

The third level of concern is mortality and its potential to reduce voter populations. Data released in 2007 by the IEC indicates that 2 679 713 registered voters died between 1999 and 2006. Monthly, South Africa loses on average 27 913 registered voters. The data also shows that the 30–39 and the 40–49 age cohorts are those most affected.

The trends in deaths among male and female voters, when aggregated, exhibit the same upward trends since 1999, with only marginal stability between 2002 and 2004. One of the key observations made in this study notes the similarities between these trends and the AIDS mortality profile described by Dorrington, et al. (2006) and WHO (2006). As in the case of councillors, many voters succumb to mortality before the age of 51. There is no new data from the IEC that informs voter mortality on the municipal rolls. Therefore no new conclusions regarding how the local authorities under study were affected by this wave of deaths can be made. Impacts on cemetery space and increased demand on clinic services might be just some of the ways attrition among VAPs will stretch the capacity of municipalities to provide services. The deaths of younger voters will also have implications for community activism. Registration should be considered a form of active citizenship, given the commitment it takes for one to volunteer to queue for registration. At a local level, these active citizens will decide who governs the community and may eventually seek political careers themselves. In general, the study could not provide a comparison of the involvement of South Africans in local government elections and their participation in subsequent by-elections, due to lack of relevant data from the IEC. The data may have demonstrated a marked difference between participation in local elections and turnout at by-elections. The analysis around the legitimacy of candidates elected into local government is, therefore, not conclusive.

THE LOCAL GOVERNMENT RESPONSE TO HIV/AIDS AND POTENTIAL FOR FRAGILITY

We also sought to understand how institutional responses by local authorities might contribute to the sustenance of municipalities' service delivery capacity by ensuring that the decision-makers and -implementers lead long, healthy lives. A poor institutional response may contribute to fragility as skilled personnel are lost regularly, undermining the local authority's capacity to deliver on the myriad demands from a restive population. Municipal managers and HIV/AIDS officers interviewed report that HIV/AIDS has increased absenteeism among all levels of staff, although this occurrence varies across municipal boundaries. A minority of these administrators noted that there had been some uptake of ARVs among office workers. Only isolated cases of councillors accessing ARVs from council clinics are cited. It cannot be inferred from available evidence that HIV/AIDS is responsible for all incidences of absenteeism, but there are consistent suggestions from the administrative staff interviewed that indicate infections within low-income grades. Although it cannot be pinned on HIV/AIDS, the description fits advancing HIV-related infections. This has key implications for productivity levels. Productivity is likely to decline as more workers are put onto lighter duties. And as key players succumb to infection, effectiveness can be expected to decline, taking along with it accountability. Many municipal areas lack an HIV policy, although their responses are guided by generic AIDS and governance frameworks advanced by the Department of Provincial and Local Government (DPLG) and SALGA. The evidence shows that the 12 municipalities have not wholly applied these frameworks due to various capacity issues. Mainstreaming – a concept promoted by the DPLG – has not been well understood. Internally, the vast majority noted the presence of Employee Assistance Programmes (EAPs) and Voluntary Counselling and Testing (VCT) initiatives. Overall, progress was regarded as inadequate as many staff members and councillors are reported to be fearful of the stigma and discrimination they would face from the wider community. The municipalities largely lack hard data, so the actual extent of impact could not be measured. Our impression is that the administrative system of local government could be as challenged by AIDS as the political system it supports, and that this may be cause for concern in terms of effectiveness of service delivery. Despite the availability of ART, pervasive denial may cause more premature deaths among elected officials and professional staff alike, contributing to weakened political and administrative systems.

CONCLUSION

Essentially, what this study does is identify weak elements in the system that may lead to fragility. This may contribute to the understanding of the issues of poor service delivery that South Africa is experiencing at local governance level. Our general impression is that the study provides not only an insight into attrition of the leadership pool and registered voters in their constituencies, it also presents a basis to interrogate further how these weaknesses relate to potential fragility in the financial and institutional systems of local government more profoundly. For instance, the frailties documented by the Auditor-General regarding the administrative and financial systems of the municipalities underline these concerns about weak governance at this level of government. Conversely, South Africa has the economic capacity to fill vacancies within its administrative system of local government ranks by importing labour from its neighbours or beyond. The government's Joint Initiative on Priority Skills Acquisition (JIPSA) strategy, adopted in 2006 as part of the Accelerated Shared Growth Initiative for South Africa (ASGISA), aimed to acquire skills for a rapidly growing economy. While the intention of JIPSA attempts to remedy national skills deficits by developing and acquiring skills, it must have 18 000 registered artisans in the 2007/08 period and about 20 000 registered artisans for the 2008/09 period for it to meet national skills needs. JIPSA must produce 50 000 artisans by 2010 for it to be considered successful.

RECOMMENDATIONS

The recommendations include a number of measures focused on: knowledge-building courses for councillors; regular medical check-ups for elected representatives to ensure early interventions and longevity; identification of champions to lead the political response; broader education around AIDS mainstreaming, accompanied by training for technical personnel. Further research is proposed on the impact of stigma and discrimination related to the uptake of ART and VCT by leaders and staff alike. Finally, a more realistic appraisal of what local government is capable of contributing to the HIV/AIDS response should be contextualised within its current capacity.

INTRODUCTION

I dasa-GAP's vision is to contribute to the building of AIDS resilient[4] democratic societies in Africa. Our mission is tailored towards the promotion of the notion of knowledgeable governance (Parsons: 1995), and the development of visionary leadership and citizen agency to deal effectively with the epidemic. The approach emphasises strong interaction between research and policy based on communicative and collaborative citizen-state relationships. Idasa-GAP aims to work through strategic policy institutions and civil society networks to bring influence to bear on national situations.

STRATEGIC APPROACHES

- Research
- Knowledge building
- Skills and leadership training

PURPOSE AND CONTEXT

Within the ASCI research agenda, this project's ambition is to respond to the need to understand 'how AIDS epidemics can contribute to state fragility' (Cluster C).

The policy goal is to enrich local authorities' responses to the epidemic by broadening the scope of knowledge and, therefore, strategic options available to mitigate impact on South African communities.

DEFINING FRAGILITY

CORE INDICATORS AND THEIR USE

Fragile states are punctuated by weak governance, institutions and policies. Indicators of fragility are framed in political, economic, social welfare and security terms (Hannan & Besada: 2007; Rice & Patrick: 2008). In order to determine the nature and extent of possible political fragility in the South African context, we shall employ three indicators from the political basket. These three indicators, which relate more closely to the role of political decision-makers are: accountability, legitimacy and effectiveness.

The study, firstly, focuses primarily on directly elected councillors who, through the lens of public opinion, appear to personify the strengths and weaknesses of local government (Bratton & Sibanyoni: 2006). Afrobarometer studies indicate that South Africans pass judgment on the efficacy of local government mainly based on the performance of their councillors, whom they expect to act as agents of change and development (ibid.). A malfunction or disruption in this representative-community relationship may have a telling impact on how matters of service delivery are perceived and how affected populations react. Although councillors are seen as 'agents of development', it stands to reason that they can only deliver if the institutions and processes supporting them, such as the local councils, are functional.

Therefore, an understanding of how the administrative system of government is affected by HIV/AIDS is relevant to the study. Similarly, understanding how the constituencies represented by councillors are affected by HIV/AIDS and their expectations on service delivery is essential, as this provides a context for the challenges decision-makers are likely to face in responding to the epidemic.

Secondly, it has to be stated that the project's ambition is not to measure fragility within the local government system in South Africa. Instead, it seeks to identify trends that may suggest the introduction of fragility over time.

Thirdly, definitions of fragility are varied, as are the means used to measure it. The presumed causes of fragility are numerous. Existing literature suggests that the concept has political, economic, security and international dimensions, among others (Hannan & Besada: 2007). Rice & Patrick (2008) observe that fragility is evaluated by four baskets of indicators which range from political and economic to security and social welfare formulations.

POLITICAL DIMENSIONS OF FRAGILITY

Rice & Patrick (2008) posit that political dimensions of fragility relate to the extent to which citizens accept their system of governance as legitimate and have regard for the quality of the state's institutions. Studies in this area will generally seek to measure the rule of law, the accountability of government to its citizens, the extent of corruption, and the ability of the state bureaucracy and institutions to perform effectively, independently and responsively. Other approaches to fragility underline humanitarian perspectives. In this case, state failure is described as a condition in which a government cannot or will not deliver on the primary social services that the majority of its people regard as their due right (Hannan & Besada: 2007).

Carment, Prest & Samy (2007) argue that state collapse is a three-stage process, which begins with the failure of government to provide adequate services to the general population. Consequently, improper channelling of resources generates ethnic, social and ideological competition, sapping the effectiveness of already weakened institutions. Lastly, the cumulative effect of poverty, overpopulation, urbanisation and rural flight, inclusive of environmental degradation, cause the state to collapse.

While there is no compelling evidence to indicate that South Africa exhibits the characteristics relating to any of these definitions, the study assumes that the complex and multisectoral nature of the HIV/AIDS epidemic can introduce indicators of fragility, particularly at a local political and administrative level. Since this study focuses on elected representatives in local government, its scope and ambition are decidedly political in nature.

We begin, therefore, by defining the three interrelated elements of fragility that make up the central themes of political fragility:

- accountability,
- legitimacy, and
- effective government.

Accountability in the context of democratic governance means that elected and public officials not only report to their superiors in the political and bureaucratic hierarchy, but also to the public. In a democracy in which accountability is upheld as a value, elected officials should ideally be responsible and answerable to the public. According to Schedler (1999:4), for example, in order for an agent to be accountable, he must be responsible or answerable to others for his decisions, and any decision he takes within the confines of legality must be enforceable.

Legitimacy is mostly understood within the Mirriam-Webster dictionary definitions as a quality that conforms to conventions. If a public representative in a democracy is to be considered legitimate, he or she must be appointed or elected within the conventions and rules regulating the processes of governance. Simmons (2000: ix–xii) suggests that legitimacy implies a popular consent that gives representatives a mandate to act.

Effectiveness is defined as a phenomenon producing a desired effect. In relation to accountability and legitimacy indicators, public representatives must consistently act within conventions and rules, and assume responsibility for the outcomes of their actions. In order for a public representative to be considered legitimate and accountable, his or her actions must promote the effective execution of the governance mandate with which he or she is entrusted. Standard usages of effective governance subsume accountability and include monitoring, performance and participation (Callahan: 2007).

The purpose of local governance in terms of political effectiveness, accountability and legitimacy can be described in the following statement:

> *The development of local democracy is essential to avoid tendencies to authoritarianism and to better meet the real needs of local people. Effective, democratic local government both delivers better local public services and gives local people a real say in the services they receive and in the way they are governed. It means that people in power locally become accountable to the people they serve, rather than to central government.* (South-East European Ministerial Conference, Zagreb: 1994)

Effective local government, as defined here, is understood as the ability of local government to represent its constituencies and deliver on the services each community considers due. In order for this to occur, local government has to be in a position to make enforceable decisions on the delivery of services. HIV/AIDS, it might be argued, has the latent potential to diminish the effectiveness of decision-making, or possibly delay it, due its debilitating nature.

The focus on the primary demographic age band (22–49) in which most skilled professionals fall suggests that councillors and skilled professionals in local government would see their numbers significantly thinned by HIV. The implication would be that South Africans would witness the replacement of skilled professionals and councillors, most likely with less-qualified and less-experienced people. In the short to medium term, a skill base of lesser quality would undermine the capacity to deliver on high-demand, essential public services. In this, the additional disruption of existing relationships between voters and elected councillors as a result of increased mortality rates, presumably due to AIDS, would reduce overall effectiveness.

Given that the public seems to conflate councillorship with service delivery, as exemplified in some Afrobarometer studies (Bratton & Sibanyoni: 2006), the absence of an elected representative in the period before by-elections are held could be perceived to contribute to ineffectiveness. In other words, the needs of the people in the affected wards might remain unheard until suitable replacements can be fielded for elections.

It can be assumed that there would be an HIV-lowered Human Development Index (HDI), with rising infections among professionals, such as teachers, engineers, town planners, accountants, health workers and managers and attrition rates among local political decision-makers, such as councillors, converging and creating the conditions of diminished effectiveness in governance. Reduced effectiveness in a resource- and capacity-stressed environment is likely to reduce the levels and realistic expectations of accountability.

Certainly, a less-qualified, inexperienced replacement cannot be realistically held to the same standards of accountability as a more capacitated participant.

Tying accountability into legitimacy is a standard frame of reference in indicators of fragility. Legitimacy and accountability may suffer if severe infection rates lead to diminishing political participation in elections and in decision-making structures. This may occur on three levels of exclusion. The first level of (self) exclusion may reside in illness-related absenteeism. Absenteeism due to HIV-related illness might also undermine effective participation by councillors in important affairs of council. A second level of exclusion may well be deliberate: those who are seen to be unwell or who publicly declare their status may run the risk of losing their claim to fresh mandates from their political parties. The third level of exclusion may be due to fatigue; voter participation in by-elections to elect new councillors may be lower than in local elections as a result of AIDS illness and care-giving commitments. One can infer this from Strand & Chirambo (2005) and Chirambo (2008), who have made the case that lower political participation can occur at the local level through illness or activities associated with caring for people falling victim to the HIV epidemic.

Strand & Chirambo (2005) assert that, while special voting mechanisms exist for national elections in South Africa, they are not extended to the local level. Stigmatisation and discrimination, a significant part of contextualising the governance aspects of this study, can further decrease the levels of social and political inclusion and participation among skilled professionals, political decision-makers and voters infected with HIV. All these features of local government's social terrain can combine to undermine the democratic experience of the governed and decrease the reinforcing relationship accountability, effective governance and legitimacy share.

TYPE OF STUDY

The larger part of the study falls squarely into the tradition described by Mouton & Marais (1996). They assert that exploratory research will not always be led by a hypothesis, but sometimes seek to cultivate the terrain of a hypothesis or many hypotheses. McNabb (2004:136–144) identifies exploratory research as a 'probing'. For McNabb, the function and purpose of exploratory research is to either engage in a preparatory examination to gather insights for future research or gather information that will be immediately applied to an administrative issue. As a result, exploratory research is generally utilised as a rapid information-gathering exercise.

Given that exploratory studies are seldom used as stand-alone methods, descriptive elements are incorporated into exploratory research to foreground and facilitate the interpretation of the data. This may be a controversial way of framing it, but, as Stebbins (2001) suggests, exploratory research is by nature controversial. However, this method may be the most effective means of providing a generic context to identifiable trends and setting out an agenda for further studies.

UNITS OF ANALYSIS

In this study, AIDS is the independent variable and the capacity of local authorities is the dependent variable. Our units of analysis are physical (councillors), institutional (municipalities, policies, practices, HIV/AIDS initiatives) and thematic (stigma and discrimination). It would not be prudent, in our view, to treat these as separate issues as they are interrelated and likely to have bearing on the whole notion of fragility.

FOCUS OF STUDY

This study uses the prism of electoral democracy to investigate the extent to which HIV/AIDS may contribute to state fragility. It seeks to determine the:
- implications of the depletion of leadership through mortality and the consequent loss of institutional memory in local government
- shifting configuration of power in local government due to by-elections and its implications for democratic accountability
- economic costs of replacing deceased councillors and sustainability of electoral models
- impact of stigma and discrimination, and functionality of leadership, at local level
- community perceptions of HIV-positive councillors and service delivery
- impact of voter mortality on political legitimacy
- local government response to HIV/AIDS and potential for fragility.

The study will finally seek to explain the ways in which the epidemic will impact on the functioning of local authorities, with all other co-factors taken into account.

METHODOLOGY

LITERATURE REVIEW

The literature review is largely framed in the 1998–2008 period, which covers the electoral cycle for local government. The period was chosen because it signifies the emergence of democratic local government in South Africa. Relevant journal articles on HIV/AIDS, reports, relevant local government legislation, books, authoritative studies on AIDS and local governance, and opinion survey data from Afrobarometer studies, were incorporated into the literature review. The rationale guiding the literature review derives from McNabb (2004), who describes this exercise in exploratory research as providing a conceptual map or the backdrop against which the issue can be understood. He suggests that the literature review can be incorporated into the technique to support it or prove the value of the data. The study relies on the assemblage of the literature review to structure and lend support to the findings.

FOCUS-GROUP DISCUSSIONS

Focus groups generally assume two generic categories: semi-structured and structured. A semi-structured focus group is guided through a moderator who initiates discussion around broadly structured questions to identify themes. A structured interview relies on the speaker guiding the conversation with a rigid question set to extract specific information (McNabb: 2004). The convened focus groups were structured along the lines of semi-structured moderation in order to identify the perceptual themes local communities have of their councillors' community roles, their ability to deliver on basic services, HIV/AIDS and development. Due to cost considerations, eight focus-group discussions were conducted across the four provinces. The rationale behind the formation of the focus groups was to aim for depth rather than quantity in understanding citizen sentiments on their councillors' performance on HIV/AIDS matters. However, we need to add a caution that these focus groups present the opinions of a small sample (74 people in total), the results of which may not have external validity. Respondents were selected from their communities, and factors such as HIV status, gender, age, level of political participation and employment status were taken into account. The urban or rural origin of the participants was also considered. Focus-group discussions were conducted in English, Afrikaans and/or African languages. To ensure the reliability of the information, participants were requested to express themselves in the language they felt most comfortable in. Translation was assured by a competent person drawn from the community.

Each of the eight discussion groups had between eight and ten respondents to ensure maximum interaction and participation. The discussion guide was loosely structured to address the following themes:
- The impact of AIDS on communities and personal experience of the epidemic.
- Knowledge of and participation in local government elections.

- Expectations and perceptions of councillors' performance.
- Voluntary Counselling and Testing (VCT) and disclosure by the leadership.
- Policy proposals on local government responses.

STATISTICAL ANALYSIS

Statistical or quantitative analysis supported the epidemiological and electoral data to determine councillor and voter attrition at ward level between 1998 and 2006, or within one complete electoral cycle. This statistical component was employed to create a national picture of local governance against which locales could be determined and compared. The resultant figures would provide a means of demonstrating the impact of HIV/AIDS on the political environment. New data was sourced on voter mortality up to 2006, against which the analysis of community-level implications were gleaned.

SEMI-STRUCTURED INTERVIEWS

Interviews were conducted with preselected councillors, HIV/AIDS officers, municipal managers and IDP managers using three questionnaires, each tailored towards the four categories of officials. A total of 112 councillors, five HIV/AIDS officers, seven municipal managers and eight IDP managers were interviewed. The councillors constituted the primary focus of the study, but in order to roughly determine the relative degree of functionality in the local councils, interviews were conducted with key local administrative staff deeply involved with HIV-planning, HIV-mainstreaming initiatives and planning, and commanding local administration. Although we could not secure interviews with all the senior management officials, each municipality presented us with an opportunity to interview either an IDP manager or a municipal manager (both functions would be privy to the same information requested in the interview questionnaires), and occasionally both. Given that there are more elected male representatives at local level than female, despite the gender parity initiatives aimed at securing an equal split of representatives on party lists, care was taken to weight the samples of representatives with a party proportionality and gender bias. An additional set of questions was targeted at the IEC with regard to by-election data, causes of vacancies and economic costs associated with by-elections.

STAKEHOLDER MEETINGS

Stakeholder meetings with key government and civil society people to discuss the findings were planned but not held due to financial limitations. They were aimed at informing the final report and, particularly, at deriving recommendations for policy directions. Dissemination of the report to selected stakeholders for comment will occur once the report is finalised.

RESEARCH LOCALITIES

It was decided to adopt an outright rural bias in our choice of research localities, since much research focus has been placed on the metropolitan structures of local government. (See, for example, Isandla's 2007 Cape Town study, Kelly's 2004 comprehensive metro study and Mathoho's 2006 Ekurhuleni metro study.) We also attempted to avoid concentrating the study in well-researched provinces such as KwaZulu-Natal (KZN), which has drawn much attention from researchers as it has the highest national HIV/AIDS antenatal average prevalence, projected to be at 40% (Dorrington, et al.: 2006). Our study examined four provinces in total: KwaZulu-Natal, Free State, Northern Cape and Western Cape.

SELECTING THE TOWNS

In each of these provinces, we chose two large towns and two smaller ones – the latter mostly within a 100 km radius of the former, often forming part of the same local government structure. In deciding on these localities, we also took into account population sizes, possible or assumed migration patterns (in itself a driver of HIV/AIDS), and known or broadly assumed poverty profiles reflected in employment data.

Table 1: Towns listed by provincial, district and municipal location			
Northern Cape	Western Cape	KwaZulu-Natal	Free State
Namakwa District Municipality • Nama Khoi Local Municipality (Springbok and Steinkopf)	**West Coast District Municipality** • Bergriver Local Municipality (Piketberg) • Saldanha Bay Local Municipality (Saldanha Bay)	**Uthukela District Municipality** • Emnambithi-Ladysmith Local Municipality (Ladysmith) • Okhahlamba Local Municipality (Bergville)	**Lejweleputswa District Municipality** • Matjhabeng Local Municipality (Welkom) • Masilonyana Local Municipality (Theunissen) • Motheo District Municipality • Mantsopa Local Municipality (Ladybrand)
Frances Baard District Municipality • Sol Plaatjie Local Municipality (Kimberley) • Magareng Local Municipality (Warrenton)		**uThungulu District Municipality** • uMhlathuze Local Municipality (Richards Bay)	**Thabo Mofutsanyane District Municipality** • Setsoto Local Municipality (Clocolan/Ficksburg)
Source: Compiled by Idasa.			

Table 2: Municipal population, prevalence and actual unemployment			
	Population (Census 2001)	Employment/ Unemployment Actual figures (age 15-65)	HIV antenatal prevalence: District level
Northern Cape			
Namakwa District			5,3%
Nama Khoi Local Municipality (Springbok and Steinkopf)	44 750	11 535 / 5 751	
Frances Baard District Municipality			22,7%
Sol Plaatjie Local Municipality (Kimberley)	201 464	46 411 / 32 927	
Magareng Local Municipality (Warrenton)	21 734	3 431 / 3 694	
Western Cape			
West Coast District			7,3%
Bergriver Local Municipality (Piketberg)	46 325	19 806 / 1 623	
Saldanha Bay Local Municipality (Saldanha Bay)	70 440	25 006 / 6 847	
KwaZulu-Natal			
Uthukela District			35,1%
Emnambithi-Ladysmith Local Municipality (Ladysmith)	225 459	42 123 / 40 857	
Okhahlamba Local Municipality (Bergville)	25 630	12 759 / 18 743	
uThungulu District Municipality			39,1%
uMhlathuze Local Municipality (Richards Bay)	289 190	67 390 / 46 065	
Free State			
Lejweleputswa District			34,1%
Matjhabeng Local Municipality (Welkom)	408 170	95 688 / 83 181	
Masilonyana Local Municipality (Theunissen)	64409	14 937 / 10 870	
Motheo District	728 263		30,5%
Mantsopa Local Municipality (Ladybrand)	55 342	12 888 / 7 097	
Thabo Mofutsanyane District	725 938		32,2%
Setsoto Local Municipality (Clocolan/ Ficksburg)	123 194	26 737 / 18 678	
Source: SSA: 2001; DoH: 2008.			

The broad rationalisations for the choices are described below:

WESTERN CAPE

On the West Coast, we chose the industrial/harbour complex of Vredenburg/Saldanha, which experiences labour migration to and from the industrial hub. It has a large fishing industry, very skewed in favour of large commercial concerns. We paired Saldanha with the small agricultural town of Piketberg.

NORTHERN CAPE

Here we selected Springbok, a large town in the north, on the N7, en route to Namibia. The area and its surrounds are dominated by the dynamics of diminishing mining activities, conflicting claims in this regard, asbestos-related illnesses and deaths, and the social and economic ramifications of communities that relied on mining as a sole source of income for decades. The 'adjacent' town we selected was Steinkopf, a desolate, small, ex-mining town, with relatively high poverty levels. Interviews here were conducted in Afrikaans. In the Northern Cape, we also chose Kimberley and its adjacent township of Galeshewe. We paired Kimberley with the small town of Warrenton, to the north.

FREE STATE

Ladybrand is the main town chosen in the eastern Free State, on the border of Lesotho. It is characterised by migration to and from Maseru, Lesotho (about 20 km away). Many people who work in Maseru live in Ladybrand and vice versa. We paired it with the small agricultural town of Clocolan, situated a relatively short distance to the north of Lady-brand. The second location was Welkom, the mining/industrial part of the Free State, where there has been generations of labour migration. We paired Welkom with the small town of Theunissen, to the south.

KWAZULU-NATAL

In KwaZulu-Natal, we selected Richards Bay/Empangeni, a relatively new industrial/harbour complex, very similar to Saldanha on the West Coast (and developed roughly at the same time and for the same reasons, about 20–30 years ago). We paired it with the small village of Gingindlovu, on the coast, to the south. We paired Ladysmith with the small town of Bergville in the Midlands. Despite strides in development over the last 15 years, KwaZulu-Natal remains a province with one of the largest HIV/AIDS-infected populations.

LIMITATIONS

Due to late availability of resources, this project essentially started at the beginning of September 2007 – not in July as originally envisaged. Despite the delays, planning sessions took place in mid-August, during which the original proposal was fleshed out, a few extra dimensions added to the study, and slight modifications to the methodology proposed and adopted. These included focus-group discussions for local community representatives, to augment the interviews with elected officials and managers.

The voter mortality data provided by the Independent Electoral Commission (IEC) only reflects national-level deaths (1999–2006). The IEC was unable to provide data up to municipal level. Without this, it is not possible for us to delve into municipal specifics in regard to mortality.

Further, municipalities do not always have hard data on staff attrition and absenteeism, and other relevant documents. In this study, and others done by Idasa, this lack of data has been raised as an issue that limits the extent to which we can quantify palpable impacts on councils and institutions.

As is to be expected, we do not have access to medical records of deceased persons and, even if we did, we would be bound by ethical considerations for non-disclosure. Hence, we rely on trend analysis: comparing age cohorts of deceased to the so-called AIDS mortality profile, from which inferences have been drawn on the main influence in deaths recorded at councillor and voter level.

The issue of language has to be considered. Most of our respondents did not use English as their first or second language. Some of the interviews were conducted in Afrikaans and translated into English. Other interviews and focus groups were conducted in local African languages and translated into English. Transcripts were assured by persons proficient in these languages.

Finally, budget limitations did not allow for the hosting of a stakeholder meeting, which had to give way to the more extensive work of actual fieldwork data-gathering. The absence of stakeholder meetings does not necessarily undermine the results; it was designed to engender 'political buy-in'. Other means of sharing the report have been devised.

REPORT ORGANISATION

The report is organised into seven chapters, in addition to this Introduction. Chapter One explicates, in great detail, the history of local government in South Africa. It explains the intricacies of amalgamation of municipal boundaries as provincial borders were re-mapped, and discusses at length the various municipal types that are in operation in the country. Distinctions are made between the administrative system and the political system, both of which are mutually reinforcing in terms of service delivery. Chapter Two addresses the notion of fragility and unpacks the basket of indicators advanced by several leading agencies before isolating the most relevant elements to this study. In this aspect of the discussion, the case is made that currently available information suggests that weaknesses in the administrative system of local governance already indicate a discernible measure of fragility.

The findings in Chapter Three unravel mortality among councillors and registered voters. It also discusses and analyses the implication for governance, and the notions of effective government, accountability and legitimacy. This chapter begins to identify some trends that may suggest fragility.

Chapters Four (stigma and discrimination), Five (community perceptions) and Six (institutional responses), continue to unfurl findings from interviews with councillors, municipal managers, HIV/AIDS officers and members of the local communities serviced by the respective municipalities. Chapter Six attempts to assess how the institutional mechanisms have responded to the varied impacts of HIV/AIDS as described in the preceding chapters. These 'coping' mechanisms will suggest whether the local response is tailored toward a holistic approach, which might absorb impacts and therefore limit the potential for fragility by extending and improving the quality of life for decision-makers and -implementers infected by HIV. General recommendations are made in the same chapter. We conclude in Chapter Seven with some reflections on the study and a discussion of potential hypotheses that might need further exploration.

CHAPTER ONE

HISTORICAL BACKGROUND OF LOCAL GOVERNMENT IN SOUTH AFRICA[5]

Until 1994, when South Africa changed to a non-racial state, local government was structured along apartheid era lines of separate development. The four large provinces – Transvaal, Natal, Cape and Orange Free State – each had an administrative system accountable to a central government with the final authority over matters of governance.

Transition from apartheid to democracy led to the enactment of a new Constitution in 1996, which set the pace for the establishment of a democratic system of local governance. While negotiations for the democratisation of national and provincial governance institutions were underway in 1993, a parallel process termed the Local Government Negotiating Forum (LGNF) was instituted to deal specifically with the complexities of local governance, leading to the Local Government Transition Act (LGTA), promulgated the same year.

The LGTA provided for a three-phase transition to local government: a pre-interim phase (1993–1995/6); an interim phase (transitional councils, pre-2000 elections); and a final phase (democratic local government, post-2000). Hence, any historical analysis of local governance in South Africa will consider the year 2000 as the critical starting point for understanding the patchwork of institutions we engage with today.

The new South Africa was sub-divided into nine provinces: Eastern Cape, Gauteng, KwaZulu-Natal, Mpumalanga, Northern Cape, Limpopo, North West, Free State and Western Cape, each with its own provincial legislature.

SEPARATION OF POWERS

The 1996 Constitution of South Africa, in Schedules 4 and 5, provides for a separation of powers and functions among central, provincial and local government. Municipalities draw their authority to preside over local matters from Section 156 of the Constitution. For strategic purposes, the Constitution also provides for cooperative governance among the three tiers in Section 41(2), to ensure the alignment of priorities, policies and activities across interrelated activities. While the national government sets the overall strategic framework for economic and social development, the provincial government is in charge of the blueprint that covers development in the province through the Provincial Growth and Development Plan (PGDP). It has the added role of ensuring that the municipal Integrated Development Plans (IDPs) are vertically integrated into the PGDP.

HOW CENTRAL GOVERNMENT LINKS WITH MUNICIPALITIES

Because of its proximity to the situation of ordinary citizens, local government in South Africa has been seen as a convergence and coordination point for programmes of other spheres of government.

STRUCTURE, POLICY AND LEGISLATION

The operational mechanism of local government in South Africa is compartmentalised into five distinct areas:
- The institutional system, which defines categories of municipalities and roles.
- The electoral system, by which council is constituted through elections
- The political system, which is the decision-making structure of the council.
- The administrative system, comprising council departments that implement decisions made by its leaders.
- Municipal finance, which comprises implementers executing decisions from the political establishment of the council.

THE INSTITUTIONAL SYSTEM

The institutional dimension breaks down municipalities into three categories:
- Metropolitan or Category A municipalities,
- Local or Category B municipalities, and
- District or Category C municipalities.

Category A (metropolitan) municipalities comprise industrial areas, business districts and relatively higher residential populations. Their financial and administrative capacities are considerable. They also tend to have only one municipal council.

Category C (district) municipalities are entities with municipal executive and legislative power in areas that contain more than one municipality. Each Category C municipality contains a number of Category B (local) municipalities. Category B municipalities are defined by viable centres of economic activity and share legislative and executive authority with Category C entities. Without a significant economic profile, Category B municipalities will be designated District Management Areas (DMAs), surrendering all authority to the Category C or district municipality (Bratton & Sibanyoni: 2006).

There are six metropolitan municipalities, 46 district municipalities and 231 local municipalities in South Africa. The six metropolitan municipalities are:
- City of Tshwane, Gauteng
- City of Johannesburg, Gauteng
- Ekurhuleni, Gauteng
- eThekwini, KwaZulu-Natal
- Nelson Mandela Metropolis, Eastern Cape
- City of Cape Town, Western Cape.

The demarcation board charged with the role of defining municipal boundaries reduced the pre-2000 profile of 844 municipal entities to 284, to ensure effective governance. As a result of the new demarcation on outer (municipal) boundaries and the delimitation of ward boundaries, the country had a total of 8 951 councillors. Of these, 3 895 were directly elected ward councillors. PR councillors stand at 5 056 (Tlakula: 2007). Following a period of amalgamation in 2005, the number of municipalities was marginally reduced to 283.

Table 3: Type and count of municipalities		
Category A	Metropolitan	6
Category B	Local	231
Category C	Districts	46

THE ELECTORAL SYSTEM

The municipalities are constituted via a Mixed Member Proportional (MMP) system, which combines the constituency-based First-Past-the-Post (FPTP) system with the Proportional Representation (PR) system. The rationale for this, it would seem, was to ensure that, at the national level, there was a deliberate effort towards broadening representation in the national and provincial legislatures, and nurturing and deepening reconciliation and political stability, while emphasising accessibility and accountability at local government levels.

The system facilitates the election of one stream of councillors through the FPTP system and the other through the PR system. In the MMP system, any disproportional representation emerging from the FPTP (or any other) system is compensated for by the PR element.

THE POLITICAL SYSTEM

The political system, the patchwork of institutional arrangements that provide for decision making, is defined in the Municipal Structures Act of 1998. The law provides for the establishment of municipalities as stipulated by the Demarcation Board. Under the Act, the Minister of Local Government and Housing is empowered to determine guidelines in assisting the Members of an Executive Committee (MECs) – the officials of provincial government – to decide which type of municipality would be appropriate for their area.

It is mandatory for each municipality to have a council that meets every quarter. The council is expected to operate in a transparent manner, but may hold sessions in camera where such action is justified. A council comprises decision makers (council committees), implementers (council departments) and the community (ward committees). There are several types of council that may be adopted:

- Mayoral Executive: The council elects an executive mayor, who then appoints members of the executive mayoral committee from the councillors who serve as his or her assistants.
- Executive Committee: An executive committee is selected by the council from among councillors, which is then mandated to elect a mayor who presides over the collective executive committee.
- Plenary Executive: The council elects its chair, the mayor, but authority is exercised in a full meeting of the council. It therefore adopts a full plenary system.

As illustrated above, the Municipal Structures Act mandates municipalities to institute a variety of political structures and assign different roles to office bearers. To fully appreciate this discussion, it is imperative that we distinctly understand the role each structure plays in the municipal superstructure.

The council, chaired by a speaker, is the legislative arm of the municipal council and is the highest decision-making body. It tables and deliberates on reports and recommendations from the mayoral executive committee and other council committees. The council may delegate certain powers and functions to other political structures, office bearers or administration for effective functioning of the municipality.

The executive mayor of the mayoral executive committee considers recommendations from council committees, maps strategic proposals to council, and monitors the management and administration of service provision to communities.

There are two types of council committees:
- Section 79 committees: The council may establish one or more committees necessary for the effective and efficient performance of any of its functions. Under this Section, the council appoints members from among councillors to determine the functions and appoint the committee chairpersons, and may authorise the committee to co-opt advisory members.
- Section 80 committees: In terms of Section 80, a municipal council with a mayoral executive committee may appoint committees of councillors to assist the mayoral executive committee. Members of the mayoral executive committee chair these types of committees.

Table 4: Differences between Section 79 and Section 80 committees

Section 79 committees	Section 80 committees
The council determines functions and may delegate powers and duties. The council appoints a chairperson. The committee may co-opt non-councillors. The committee is established for the effective performance of functions of the council.	The executive mayor delegates powers and duties. The executive mayor appoints a chairperson. The committee only consists of councillors. The committee is established to assist the executive mayor.
Source: Johannesburg Council: 2004.	

Council committees can also be categorised as:
- portfolio committees
- geographically based committees, and
- issue-related committees.

THE ADMINISTRATIVE SYSTEM

The notion of developmental local government – a product of the Constitution and the White Paper on local government – defines a vision of close collaboration between municipalities and communities to achieve sustainable human development. The key elements of developmental local government are:

- Enhancing social development and economic growth. Municipalities are expected to focus on cost-effective, affordable delivery of basic services.
- Integration and coordination. Through the IDPs, municipalities are expected to lead and coordinate all stakeholders toward developmental goals.
- Democratising development. Municipalities must ensure that all people participate in decisions affecting their welfare.
- Leading and learning. Municipalities should have the ability to learn from global partners, strategise, develop visions and policies, and mobilise resources in line with developmental blueprints.

The instruments and methods that can be utilised by local government to achieve the ambitions of this developmental role include:

- integrated development planning and budgeting,
- performance management and monitoring, and
- working with local citizens and partners.

Among other things, a legal framework for local public administration and human resource development governs the administrative systems. That framework also seeks to empower the poor and ensure that municipalities institute service tariffs, credit control and debt-collection policies responsive to their needs, and formulate a framework for the provision of services, service-delivery agreements and municipal service districts.

Administrative systems are also designed to establish an enabling mechanism to facilitate planning, performance management, resource mobilisation and organisational change, which buttress the concept of developmental local government.

MUNICIPAL FINANCE

Financial management systems within individual municipalities are expected to provide an integrated approach for managing municipal finances, enabling effective control, accountability, monitoring and evaluation. The institutional arrangement giving impetus to developmental local government is the IDP. In terms of the Local Government Municipal Act of 2000, all municipalities are required to prepare IDPs to guide their business.

These five-year strategic plans are reviewed annually in consultation with communities and stakeholders. IDPs aim to achieve service delivery and development goals for municipal areas in an effective and sustainable way. National and provincial sector departments, development agencies, private sector bodies, NGOs and communities all have key and supportive roles to play in the preparation and implementation of municipal IDPs.

The structures and the prescribed, cooperative nature of the three tiers of government in South Africa all provide an apparently strong basis for dealing with the challenges of underdevelopment.

CHAPTER TWO

THE PROBLEM: POTENTIAL FOR FRAGILITY IN LOCAL GOVERNMENT

Fourie (2003) suggests that nations in Sub-Saharan Africa are not directly headed for state failure. Indeed, while threats may be underestimated in this view, we suggest that it would take a while for HIV/AIDS to filter its way into the democratic process. Rice & Patrick (2008) define the condition of state fragility thus:

> …[S]uch countries lack the capacity and/or will to perform core functions of Statehood effectively. In other words, weak States are unable or unwilling to provide essential public services, which include fostering equitable and sustainable economic growth, governing legitimately, ensuring physical security, and delivering basic services. (2008:5)

This obviously occurs within the bounds of the myriad definitions informing state fragility, which is measured differently depending on the functions of state that are emphasised.

The Center for Global Development (CGD) measures fragile or weak states on the basis of capacity, legitimacy and security. Only one indicator – childhood immunisation, accountability and battle deaths respectively – is used to measure each field. No overall list of ranked weak states emerges from their system of fragility measurement.

The Department for International Development (DFID) defines fragility according to a series of indicators measuring the state's will and capacity to use domestic and international resources to deliver security, social welfare, economic growth and legitimate political institutions. As with the CGD, no relative picture emerges from their ranking system.

The United States Agency for International Development (USAID) measures economic, political, social and security spheres using 33 indicators to determine the degree of fragility. They concede, however, that state 'effectiveness' and 'legitimacy' do not always carry a consistent view of fragility. It appears hence that legitimacy and effectiveness do not necessarily lend mutual support in determining fragility, making it difficult to measure with precision.

Of all the indicators used to measure fragility, the following four generic categories – economic, security, social welfare and political – appear to be common to all measuring criteria (see, for example, USAID: 2005; DFID: 2005).

- Economic indicators of fragility cover income inequality, inflation, the quality of regulation, Gross Domestic Product (GDP) growth and Gross National Income (GNI) per capita.
- Security issues are covered by the indicators of conflict intensity, human rights abuses, territory afflicted by conflict, incidences of coups and the stability of political outcomes indicated by the absence of violence.
- Social welfare indicators cover child mortality, access to basic services such as sanitation and water, degree of undernourishment in the population and life expectancy.
- Political indicators cover government effectiveness, rule of law, accountability, corruption control measures and freedom. This is the basket of indicators that we have found directly relevant to political decision-making and project implementation at local level.

CAPACITY ISSUES IN LOCAL GOVERNMENT

It has to be stated at the outset that, even without AIDS, the ambitions of local government in South Africa since 1993 appeared compromised by a myriad capacity-related issues.

In 2002, the government of South Africa realised that the newly amalgamated and reconstructed municipalities lacked the technical capacities to deal with the growing demands of service delivery from previously disadvantaged communities.

Health, water and sanitation, spatial land management and social services were some of the problem areas that municipalities grappled with. Government also noted issues associated with the uncoordinated devolution of powers and functions of local government in relation to national and provincial government (Project Consolidate: 2004).

To address the issue, the government launched 'Project Consolidate', crafted at the ministerial level, which emphasised interdepartmental cooperation. Project Consolidate aimed to tackle the backlogs in service delivery apparent in the most under-developed municipalities (DPLG: 2007). Provincial human development indicators (SSA: 2006) show that municipalities selected for capacity building also manifested the lowest human development rankings.

Project Consolidate defined the core mandate of local government thus:

a   Public participation, ward committees and community development workers
b   Human relations posture and electoral administration
c   Indigent policy, free basic services, billing systems and municipal debt
d   Expanded public works programme, Municipal Infrastructure Grant (MIG) and Local Economic Development (LED)
e   Anti-corruption
f   Special interventions
g   Performance management framework, indices and communication.

(Project Consolidate: 2004)

In its review of 2004, the project revealed that municipalities were not institutionally prepared to perform their traditional local government functions of providing water and sanitation services, and other related tasks. What is noticeable by its absence from the 2004/2006 Project Consolidate document, is HIV/AIDS as a significant factor that may undermine the sustainability of local government. The epidemic was not defined in Project Consolidate as a core integrated part of municipal business (DPLG: 2007).

This might be reflective of the rather undecided approach that the government adopted toward redressing the epidemic after 1994. It is worth noting that, given the government assessment, many municipalities participating in Project Consolidate did not have sufficient capacity to drive service delivery and, by implication, were not in a position to shoulder the added mandate of responding to HIV/AIDS.

While Project Consolidate does not foreground HIV/AIDS as an integral part of local government, we later find the government shores up this initiative with the 2007 Department of Provincial and Local Government (DPLG) framework on AIDS and governance. Project Consolidate was conceived as a temporary measure, so funding for the programme may not extend beyond 2008. It is hence logical to assume that if local government struc-tures do not meet the standard required of their developmental mandates, the newer framework of the DPLG may not be fully and functionally implemented.

Documenting the shift from Project Consolidate criteria to the DPLG's mainstreaming policy helps us to contrast policy framework shifts. The newer of the policies, the DPLG framework for local governance, comprises eight pillars, which interface with HIV/AIDS in all spheres:

- Legislative compliance: Ensure that all municipalities understand and fulfil their constitutional and legal obligations with regard to HIV/AIDS, and implement rel-evant governance and development responses.
- Equal access: Promote universal distribution of services and the availability of adequate housing and sanitation, food security, safe and affordable water and power supply, good roads and transportation, especially for HIV-infected and -affected individuals in all municipalities.
- Equity: Ensure equitable distribution of services in a manner that is non-discrimi-natory across individuals infected or affected by HIV, and those not infected or affected by HIV/AIDS, in all municipal areas.
- Flexibility: Adopt a differentiated approach that determines current response lev-els, builds on strengths, and tailor-make interventions to meet local needs.
- Incrementalism: Roll out support in a progressive manner over time.
- Capacity building and leadership: Promote and develop appropriate competencies among all role players to carry out their responsibilities in responding to the HIV/AIDS challenge.
- Partnerships: Facilitate comprehensive stakeholder consultations and dialogue, encouraging partnership-driven development in planning and implementation of relevant HIV/AIDS responses involving all spheres of government, civil society, the private sector and development agencies.
- Human rights based approach: Promote the protection of human rights and dignity of HIV-affected and -infected individuals.

(DPLG: 2007:12)

The DPLG framework presents a relatively holistic HIV/AIDS approach to local au-thorities and advances the notion of mainstreaming succinctly. It encourages internal and external assessment of the impact of HIV/AIDS on local authorities, and favours cross-sectoral involvement in strategies.

The South African Local Government Association (SALGA) (2008) provides perhaps an even more simplified reflection of what constitutes mainstreaming in the context of local government. Building on the emerging notion of governance and AIDS, the docu-ment presents a blueprint with six main components informed by the Alliance of Mayors Initiative for Community Action on AIDS at the Local Level (AMICALL). The key ele-ments are:

- promoting an effective leadership response for HIV/AIDS,
- enhancing local government input into policy development,
- increasing local capacity for an effective internal response,
- increasing local capacity for an effective external response,

- promoting partnerships, and
- ensuring implementation, monitoring and sustainability.

The blueprint goes further and advises local authorities on how to link each area of operation with HIV/AIDS. Essentially, the framework places HIV/AIDS as a core activity in any form of planning undertaken by local authorities. Table 5 shows the range of holistic interventions that local authorities are advised to undertake.

Table 5: Mainstreaming at the local government level	
Administrative services	Ensure that non-discrimination policies are implemented and monitored in all areas of local government work.
Water and waste services	IDPs that have a bias to providing basic services such as water and sanitation.
Road and transport infrastructure and services	Ensure that road infrastructure projects prioritise access to facilities such as clinics, hospitals and identified home-based care centres.
Refuse removal and storm water management systems	Ensure that there is a system for safe disposal of needles and sharps, as well as medical waste.
Municipal transport	Route plans that are friendly; public transport stops provided with shelters
Land/buildings for residential, business or other uses, such as burial grounds	Address the growing need for burial plots within the planning of land uses.
Disaster management	In designing temporary accommodation for people displaced by disaster, the layout should take care to reduce the rape risk for women and girls.
Libraries, parks, sport and recreation	Integrate HIV/AIDS awareness and anti-stigma into public leisure events.
Source: SALGA: 2008.	

This framework, at least in principle, underlines the need for planners, engineers, accountants, administrators and political leaders to account for HIV/AIDS in all of their policy inputs and day-to-day functions. Conversely, we can also understand this presentation as recognising that HIV/AIDS is not simply an issue of health, but one that requires a multifaceted approach, with a rights-driven coordinated approach at policy, institutional and community levels. The framework, however, assumes that local authorities are fully equipped in terms of human and financial resources to be able to drive a mainstreamed strategy of this scale.

The experiences of 2008 when disadvantaged communities took to the streets disaffected by lack of service delivery underline this persistent perception of weak governance. With the ravages of HIV/AIDS, communities are likely to constantly knock on the doors of their representatives seeking AIDS relief, among other things. Ironically, AIDS appears to gradually present itself as one of the key factors causing worker attrition and possibly also affecting service delivery (Isandla: 2007).

Essentially, research addresses the weaknesses of the administrative system or the implementing wing of local government (see Whiteside & Sunter: 2000; Isandla: 2007). When mixed with possible weaknesses in the political system of local government, this scenario begins to suggest a rather ominous picture of potential declines in effectiveness in governance. Increasing ineffectiveness in governance would raise the potential HIV/AIDS has to undermine the state's ability to positively act on the issues of economic management, to preserve the stability of political outcomes and to deliver basic services. Hence, effective government directly feeds into the fragility debate.

The Human Development Report (2000) suggests that HIV/AIDS is beginning to reverse the general quality of life for the South African people. The decline of the state's ability to provide basic services and to create self-generative and transferable human capital, as evidenced in the Human Development Index (HDI) projections for the last 12 years, is directly attributable to HIV/AIDS.

Table 6: Projected HDI for South Africa (1996–2008)		
Year	Without AIDS	With AIDS
1996	0.628	0.626
1997	0.628	0.624
1998	0.644	0.619
1999	0.645	0.612
2000	0.646	0.605
2001	0.647	0.597
2002	0.648	0.589
2003	0.648	0.580
2004	0.649	0.572
2005	0.650	0.565
2006	0.651	0.559
2007	0.651	0.554
2008	0.652	0.549
Source: SA UNDP Human Development Report (2000).		

What makes the downward trend in human development noticeably ominous is that the majority of people infected with HIV/AIDS are in the most economically active age cohort. Of the 5,4 million infected in South Africa, 18,8% are economically available and active adults aged between 15 and 49 (Dorrington, et al.: 2006).

Across communities, the HIV/AIDS epidemic is reducing life expectancy, increasing infant mortality, fuelling poverty, and generating a greater need for health care and state aid. At the same time, available resources are stretched, sectors of the economically active population have been dying, existing social and economic inequalities are being compounded, and the number of orphans and vulnerable persons requiring state aid and care have continued to multiply (Whiteside & Sunter: 2000: World Bank: 2003; Swartz & Roux: 2004).

Estimates made in 2006 indicate that over 1,5 million South African children have been maternally orphaned by AIDS. These children are now dependent on grants, state care and relatives (Dorrington, et al.: 2006). It is further suggested that rising incidences of AIDS-illnesses – 599 298 AIDS-sick by mid-2006 in South Africa alone (ibid.) – may cause the demand for state resources to outstrip the capacity of the state to supply them. In addition, AIDS-affected households would be unable to service household debt, pay municipal rates or engage in taxable economic activity. Not only would these inabilities undercut state organ revenue bases, but also negatively influence national economic health.

Overall, declining human development indices increase the social responsibilities of government and add to the taxation and social responsibilities of the economically engaged. Additionally, the skills pool from which the government can draw to populate its functions is likely to decrease as the levels of technically able and economically active are reduced through HIV/AIDS. The combined effect of attrition of skilled and semi-skilled personnel and the needs of the communities are likely to stretch the resources available to local government to dangerously destabilising levels.

Without adequate funding and with the constellation of new contending social and governance priorities introduced by HIV/AIDS, the greater roles expected of local government in regard to improving the health of citizens, and providing housing, water and land resources, will not be easily attainable.

Research around local government and HIV/AIDS has not explored the consequences borne by local authorities when elected leaders and other decision makers succumb to disease; and how this might further compound the perceptions of ineffectiveness at this level.

FRAGILITY EMERGING AT COUNCILLOR LEVEL?

In this regard, it is important to note that Project Consolidate recognised as far back as 2004 that there was a public 'perception that some councillors are unable to provide assistance to communities, with the smallest of their problems' (Project Consolidate: 2006: 8). Among other things, the project sought to build capacity for better accountability by public representatives, with regular interaction between councillors and the communities through 'one-stop' government centres and *Imbizos* (public policy forums).

The initiatives recognised that there were major challenges associated with:
- the wide demarcation of ward boundaries and the need for creative solutions,
- limited funds for the operation of ward committees,
- administrative demands on councillors' time, with implications on direct contact with households and communities,
- low voter turnout,
- councillor accountability, and
- citizen knowledge of rights.

In terms of the government's 2004 electoral mandate, and its 2000 local government electoral mandate, there is an obligation by government to ensure that councillors are committed and accountable to their communities. To enforce this, the electoral mandate requires that all councillors sign a code of conduct requiring them to report back to their constituencies; fight corruption in tendering, hiring and other government functions; and declare all their assets and business interests. However, there is also recognition that there is some discontent with councillors (ibid.: 11).

Popular discontent with delivery suggests that these initiatives are not as effective as communities would like. South Africa has seen dissatisfied populations take to the streets demanding the delivery of basic services to their communities. Riots and open clashes between members of communities, such as Khutsong (near Johannesburg), a community rejecting redrawn municipal boundaries, and the police have generated much debate and media coverage. The wave of xenophobic attacks, which culminated in mob-style murders, arson and theft in Alexandra, Primrose and Diepsloot in Gauteng, are largely speculated to be linked to disaffection with service delivery, among other issues (*The Star*: 20/05/2008, 21/05/2008). This phenomenon has reared its head largely among historically disadvantaged communities, particularly the black population in South Africa, who continue to raise concerns about the performance of local government.

Notwithstanding the prospect that the roles and responsibilities of councillors may be ill-understood by their constituencies, the blame seems to lie squarely at the elected officials' doorstep. We infer from these developments and from Afrobarometer public opinion surveys that councillors are seen as agents of change/development as well as local legislators. The adult population of South Africa would hence expect their material well-being to be advanced by the councillors whom they elect every five years through the Mixed Member Proportional (MMP) system. The roles and responsibilities of municipal councillors in South Africa are embedded in several pieces of legislation. However, the specific role of councillors is in the Municipal Systems Act 2000, in Schedule 1 on the code of conduct for councillors, which states:

> *Councillors are elected to represent local communities on municipal councils, to ensure that municipalities have structured mechanisms of accountability to local communities, and to meet the priority needs of communities by providing services equitably, effectively and sustainably within the means of the municipality. In fulfilling this role, councillors must be accountable to local communities and report back at least quarterly to constituencies on council matters, including the performance of the municipality in terms of established indicators.*

Given this description, public expectations of their local representatives may be assessed, to some extent, within the bounds of reality.

To fully appreciate this discussion on public perception, we again turn to the Afrobarometer studies, which show that just under half of South Africa's adult population believe local government is working well (Bratton & Sibanyoni: 2006). The levels of satisfaction are lower among rural folk than urban populations. Black people are the least satisfied of the races. The study shows that all South Africans judge local government performance in terms of their perceptions of whether the elected councillor is doing a good job.

Bratton & Sibanyoni (2006) underline this impression in their study. They assert that Africans relate democratisation to socio-economic delivery. In South Africa, historically disadvantaged communities view democratic reforms as a means to ending economic and social exclusion institutionalised by apartheid. Afrobarometer expects that confidence levels in local government will decline over time. While conceding that the period 2004–2006 was too short to anticipate any significant trends, the study shows that the number of South Africans who believe the government is handling affairs well at local level is in decline.

Figure 1: Popular assessments of local government performance in 2004 and 2006

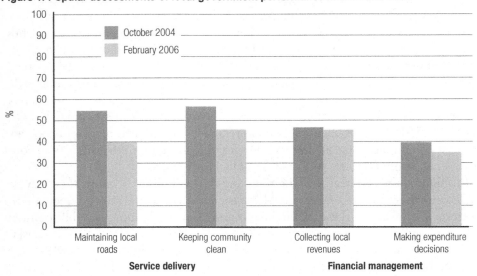

Source: Bratton and Sibanyoni (2006).

The largest declines were recorded for service delivery. Satisfaction with road mainte-nance, for instance, declined 15 points from 56% in 2004 to 41% in 2006. An 11-point decline was registered for refuse collection over the same period.

Downward trends were also registered for fiscal performance. Bratton & Sibayoni (2006) attribute this apparent decline in confidence to four factors:

- The postponement of local elections from early 2005 to March 2006, which pro-jected a sense of disorganisation.
- Political protests at lack of service delivery punctuated low-income townships of key metropolitan municipalities, including those in Gauteng, Durban and Cape Town in the 2004–2006 period. The wide media coverage was taken as a measure of mass discontent with the performance of incumbent political leaders.
- Media reported prominent cases of corruption regarding housing and local govern-ment programmes in Matjhabeng and Phomolong, Free State.
- Service delivery deficits took centre stage in the local government election cam-paigns in 2006.

There are variations across provinces in terms of satisfaction levels, but the four prov-inces without metropolitan councils – Mpumalanga, Limpopo, North West and Northern Cape – reported the highest dissatisfaction.

On the contrary, the four provinces with metro councils – Gauteng, KwaZulu-Natal, Eastern Cape and Western Cape – indicate satisfaction with the delivery of public services. Afrobarometer explains these variances as emanating from a number of factors:

- Demographic factors, where people's assessment is based on their social back-ground. Hence urban whites are deemed to be more positively inclined than his-torically disadvantaged, rural blacks.

Figure 2: Popular service delivery assessment

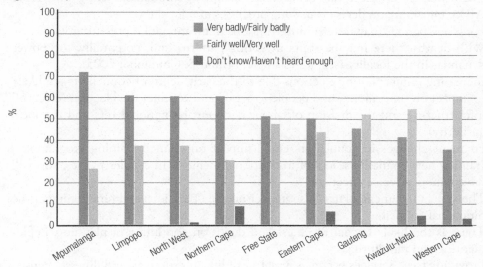

Source: Bratton and Sibanyoni (2006).

- Individual attitudes. All individuals are rational beings who decide whether their council or councillor is performing based on their personal experience of the world around them.
- The most critical factor, they assert, is whether people think their councillor is doing a good job.

This last factor is so influential, the study reports, as to cause people to make positive or negative judgement of the performance of the entire system of local government (Bratton & Sibanyoni: 2006: 12). Afrobarometer concludes that South Africans experience political authority directly and intimately through the functions of local government characterised by the payment of annual property rates and monthly household bills. Government performance is experienced through the provision of basic and social services, the absence of which may lead to negative judgement on performance (Ibid.: 14).

The rise in HIV/AIDS infections may complicate this scenario by causing the very people in whom public trust resides to neglect their mandates due to illness, to be reluctant to attend public engagements if they are emaciated, and to be unable to respond to the immediate needs of the constituencies if constantly ill.

Their effectiveness may not only be undermined in this regard, but they may also be deemed to be unaccountable to the populations that voted them in. Given that restive rural populations have already demonstrated some elements of dissatisfaction across South Africa, we cannot possibly underestimate the plausibility of these arguments. Deaths that regularly cause wards to go unrepresented may present an even more frustrating situation for the mass of expectant people. Few would turn up to vote in subsequent by-elections due to a myriad reasons: fatigue, illness, care-giving, job-seeking, or prioritising issues of survival. In summary, the large number of people infected with HIV/AIDS is especially significant to local democracy in several ways:

- There may be erratic levels of productivity among councillors living with HIV/AIDS, impacting on decision-making processes at a local level
- Long sick periods may result in interruptions in meaningful representivity.
- With deaths, there may be shifts in voting patterns and, potentially, the power dynamics in the locality (see, for example, Strand & Chirambo: 2005).
- Increasing numbers of by-elections due to the early death of councillors are likely to impact on time, money and people to set up and conduct the election (electoral infrastructure and the division of labour between the national IEC and the local authority).
- Frequent changes in councillors could impact on council training programmes, training new councillors, loss of institutional memory. In smaller parties, this will have a more adverse effect.
- The shifts in councillors may also impact on the operations and functioning of the municipal council.
- There is the likely impact of illness and death on continuity of planning, implementing and monitoring.
- Providing basic services becomes a matter of life and survival, and illnesses caused by HIV/AIDS decrease the ability of affected households to pay for these essential services.
- There are fewer income-generating options for people who fall ill with opportunistic infections.
- Transient populations and migratory labour hinder the capacity of municipalities to plan properly and may create fluctuations in community service demands.

In Chapter Three we begin to unravel mortality among ward councillors and their communities, particularly registered voters in South Africa, in order to glean some understanding of what the governance implications might be and how they may be dealt with. The chapter places mortality within the context of fragility by relating its findings to the three key indicators: effectiveness, accountability and legitimacy.

CHAPTER THREE

FINDINGS: IMPACT OF AIDS ON THE POLITICAL SYSTEM

W e indicated earlier that the political system of local government in South Africa is defined in the Municipal Structures Act of 1998, and is characterised by a variety of municipal types: mayoral executive, executive committee and plenary executive. Decision-makers who are either directly elected or proportionally allocated to their seats, essentially inhabit these structures.

In this study we concentrate on the directly elected representatives who number 3 895 out of 8 951 councillors (the balance of whom are assigned through proportional representation). We also analyse mortality among registered voters, attempt to understand how wards may be affected in terms of available active participants in public processes (such as elections), and in what ways political decision-makers will be challenged to deal with the matter.

The means by which we track attrition among directly elected councillors is through the causes of by-elections. It has to be reiterated that we do not have access to confidential records on the actual causes of deaths among ward councillors, which limits our ability to categorically attribute mortality to AIDS. However, we do rely on inferences based on the following approaches:

- We analyse the ages of councillors. Where there is a preponderance of deaths among councillors below age 49, inferences may be drawn on the possible causes of such a mortality profile.
- We compare the trends in deaths to AIDS mortality in the general population. Is there a correspondence in patterns?
- We locate the deceased in their respective provinces. Are the majority located in provinces with double-digit HIV/AIDS prevalence rates?

CAUSES OF ATTRITION AMONG WARD COUNCILLORS

The data suggests that out of 589 by-elections held between 28 February 2001 and December 2007 nationwide, 285 were caused by the deaths of ward councillors. Some 241 by-elections were caused by councillors resigning their positions, 44 were dismissed, five expelled and two imprisoned, resulting in further by-elections during the same period.

While there is no indication that these deaths resulted from shootings, accidents or disease, the first impression is that death is the leading cause of vacancies among directly elected councillors in South Africa. The deaths occurred mostly within a single electoral cycle.

Death accounts for 48,7% of all vacancies, compared to resignation at 40,9%, termination of councillor membership by party at 7,5%, dissolution of council by MEC 2%, expulsions 0,8%, and imprisonment 0,1%.

Figure 3: By-election justification (2001–2007)

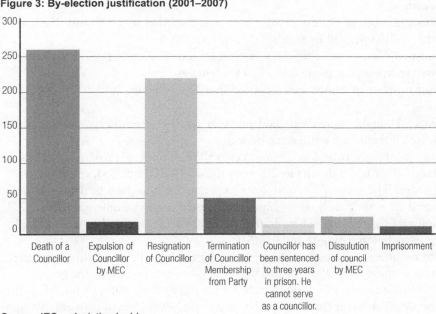

Source: IEC; calculation by Idasa.

DECEASED COUNCILLORS BY GENDER

When broken down by gender per year, the mortality data shows that more male councillors died than female councillors between 2001 and 2007. In total, 217 male councillors died from undisclosed causes during this period, compared to 54 women. This is likely due to the fact that the majority of the councillors are male.

Figure 4: Disaggregated councillor deaths (2001–2007)

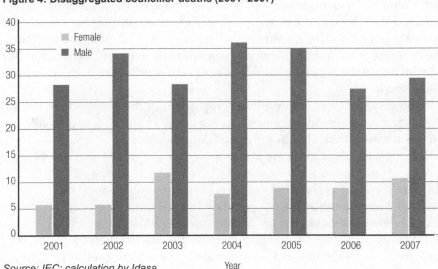

Source: IEC; calculation by Idasa.

Other observations are:

- The highest number of deaths among men was recorded in 2004 and 2005, the period when AIDS peaked in South Africa (DoH: 2006).
- The highest female mortality figures were recorded in 2003 and 2007. Deaths fluctuated over the years but peaked in 2003 for females.
- The lowest number of deaths was recorded in 2006 for males, and 2001 and 2002 for females.
- On average, 31 male councillors died per year for the seven years, compared to eight female councillors for the same period.

In 2001 alone, local authorities lost 28 male councillors. This figure rose to 34 in 2002, and then declined by six to 28 deaths in 2003. In the 2004–2005 period, the number of deaths peaked at 36. The years 2006 and 2007 experienced a decline in deaths among males aged 27 and 29 respectively. By comparison, deaths among women in 2001/2002 remained constant at five deaths. They doubled in 2003 and stabilised at around eight deaths for three years before rising to ten in 2007.

The absolute numbers, as already indicated, do not explain the possibility that there may have been more male councillors or female councillors in a particular age group.

We cannot state the rate at which deaths are increasing or decreasing. A related point is that there is no information at this stage on the total number of elected men and women in the local authority establishment in general for the years 2001 to 2007. It may well be that, in relative terms, the percentage of women who died in each of those years was far higher than that of men.

DECEASED FEMALE COUNCILLORS BY AGE

One of our key concerns in this study is to determine whether the elected leaders who are deceased fall in the older age band (i.e. 50 years and above) or whether they fall in the 20–49 age group, which has been assessed to be most vulnerable to HIV/AIDS.

We have indicated that this is the age group that is likely to constitute the core of the economically active population. The age variable allows us to infer whether the majority, if not all, of the deceased were in the advanced stages of their lives and were naturally poised to die, in which case the argument for AIDS as a possible influence in these deaths might be extremely weak.

Conversely, if the majority, or certainly a large proportion, of the deceased are below the age of 50, we may strengthen our arguments in respect of HIV/AIDS and its role in these deaths. In this regard, the gender-disaggregated data shows that:

- deaths among female councillors are concentrated in the 40–44 and 45–49 age groups,
- no deaths were recorded in the 20–24 age group for the seven years,
- only one death occurred in the 60–64 age group in 2007, and
- only one death was recorded in the 65–69 age group in 2004.

Eight women councillors in the 35–39 age cohort died in the 2001–2007 period, 17 in the 40–44 age group and nine in the 45–49 segment. There were no deaths among

Figure 5: Female councillor mortality (2001–2007)

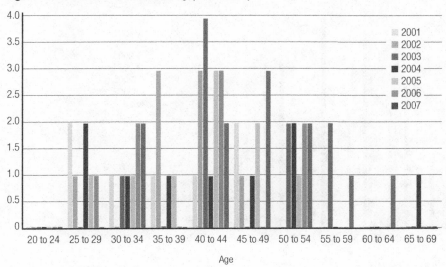

Source: IEC; calculations by Idasa.

women over the age of 50 years in the period 2001–2002. Over the seven years, the local authorities lost only three women aged 55–59 years. There were virtually no deaths in the 60–64 age group for six years, until 2007, when one female councillor died. Similarly, only one woman between the ages of 65-69 died in the seven-year period.

This may be explained by the possibility that there are relatively few councillors in the 65–69 age group, or that, if their numbers are significant, they would be in relatively good health and therefore not dying at the same rate as those in other age groups. Similarly, there may have been fewer councillors over the age of 55. Ultimately, it may also be suggestive of their belonging to ethnic groups that are less susceptible to HIV/AIDS.

DECEASED MALE COUNCILLORS BY AGE

The data shows that male deaths totalled 217. In 2001, male councillors in the 35–39 and 25–29 age groups accounted for 21% of all the deaths among this gender; while the 60–64 age cohort accounted for only 3,4%. The largest number of councillors to die came from the 45–49 age group and accounted for 23% of deaths. Other salient observations include the following:

- There were fewer deaths in the 20–24; 60–64 and 65–69 age groups.
- The highest number of deaths was in the 30–34 age group in 2002.
- Deaths among the 40–44 age cohort peaked in 2004.
- Since 2005, no deaths have been recorded for the 60–64 and the 65–69 age groups.

This might be explained by the possibility that there was no one in the 60–69 age group serving as a councillor in local government in that particular year, or that the councillors in that age group did not succumb to either natural or unnatural deaths.

Figure 6: Male councillor mortality (2001–2007)

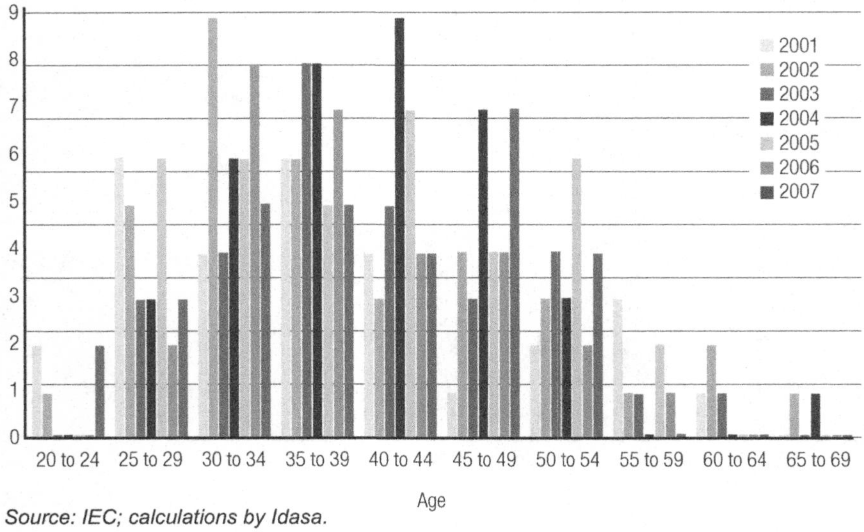

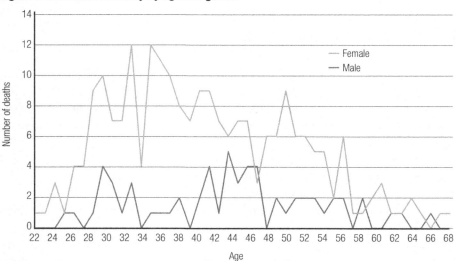

Source: IEC; calculations by Idasa.

MALE AND FEMALE DECEASED COUNCILLORS COMPARED

There is no distinct pattern emerging when male and female deaths are compared. Female mortality patterns are characterised by regular fluctuations. While there are no corresponding patterns in general between the two data sets, we do note that there is a concentration of deaths in both sexes in the economically active population aged 29-42.

The most important observation from the graph is that the majority of South African councillors who have died have done so before reaching age 51.

Figure 7: Councillor mortality by age and gender

Source: IEC; calculations by Idasa.

LIFE EXPECTANCY AND ART

The age profile of deceased councillors is highly unusual in a healthy population, which tends to have more deaths upward of age 50 years (Strand & Chirambo: 2005). World Health Organisation (WHO) statistics on average life expectancy in South Africa indicate that South Africans will die before reaching the average age of 51 (WHO: 2006).

Figure 8: Average life expectancy country comparison (2004)

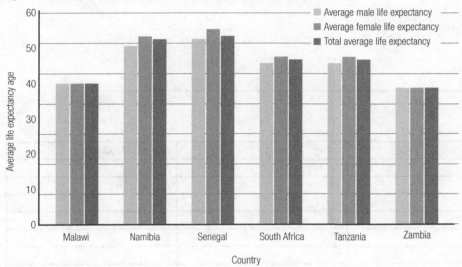

Source: WHO: 2006.

Dorrington, et al. (2006) underline this by asserting that AIDS has subtracted 13 years off the life expectancy of South Africans, reducing it from 64 years to 51 years. The mortality profile described by WHO (2006) and Dorrington, et al. (2006) certainly reflect similarities in the trends in deaths observed among ward councillors in South Africa. In the age of treatment, it is suggested that South Africans will live longer. Dorrington, et al. (2004) also indicate that 70% of all deaths in 2004 in the 15–49 age group were due to AIDS. The figure declined to 45% when all adults (15+) were factored in. If these statistics were taken as a constant over the 2001–2007 period, we could assume that 70% of the councillors in South Africa died of AIDS. However, this would require us to make further assumptions:

- Councillors are universally representative of all South Africans.
- Gender of the councillors is of a representative parity.
- A constant AIDS death ratio applies to all of South Africa for the period 2001–2007.
- An even distribution of HIV/AIDS prevails across the entire country.

Based on this reasoning, Figure 9 shows that 70% of mortality among councillors in the 22–49 age group is attributable to AIDS. In other words, using this logic, 163 councillors would have died of AIDS.

Figure 9: Councillor mortality with 70% AIDS ratio factored in (22–49 years)

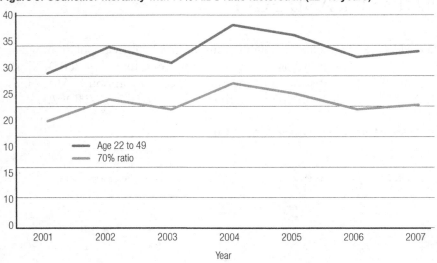

Year	Count	70% HIV/AIDS ratio
2001	29	20
2002	34	24
2003	31	22
2004	38	27
2005	36	25
2006	32	22
2007	33	23
Total	233	163
Source: IEC; Dorrington, et al. (2004); calculations by Idasa.		

IMPACT OF ANTI-RETROVIRAL THERAPY

Dorrington, et al. (2006) suggest further that, without a treatment programme, the average life expectancy will drop to 48 years by 2015. With an Anti-retroviral Therapy (ART) programme, however, the average life expectancy would be 50 years.

In their report on the potential impact of ART, they further project that, by 2010, AIDS deaths per annum will fall from 505 000 to 388 000. Deaths would fall to 291 000 if 90% of all in need of ART were to access it (ibid.).

Councillors have a relatively higher standard of living than ordinary members of the community. The municipal councils surveyed in this study all suggest they have medical aid schemes for all staff and that councillors may choose to enlist with their schemes.

While there was no hard data on the extent to which ART has been accessed by councillors and staff, there are indications from municipal managers that some degree of usage has occurred.

COUNCILLORS: REFLECTING ON THE IMPACT OF HIV/AIDS

The personal experience of councillors expressed in this study, though guarded, also resonates with the possible conclusion of AIDS as one, if not the main, cause of the larger proportion of deaths.

Although our study shows that there is a general reluctance among councillors to disclose their HIV status, they present a fairly strong impression of how the elected representatives have experienced HIV/AIDS. Some 59,4% of respondents said they had lost a family member, relation or friend to AIDS; 16,8% said they knew a fellow councillor/s that had died of the disease.

Examined at a municipal level, the responses still project a fairly solid impression of the impact of AIDS on the personal lives of councillors, with the exception of four areas: 16,6% in Ladysmith/Bergville, 75% in Richards Bay, 20,7% in Welkom/Theunissen and 10% in Ladybrand/Clocolan/Ficksburg said they knew fellow councillors who had died of AIDS. By contrast, councillors in Springbok/Steinkopf, Piketberg/Saldanha and Kimberley/Warrenton said they did not know of any fellow councillor who had died of AIDS.

Table 7: Councillor knowledge of HIV/AIDS attrition expressed as a percentage		
	Loss of family/relative/friend	Loss of colleagues/councillors
Expressed as percentage of total	59,4%	16,8%
Springbok/Steinkopf	42%	0
Piketberg/Saldanha	42%	0
Ladysmith/Bergville	61%	16,6%
Richards Bay	75%	75%
Kimberley/Warrenton	25%	0
Welkom/Theunissen	72,4%	20,7%
Ladybrand/Clocolan/Ficksburg	65%	10%
Source: Field data.		

IMPACT OF COUNCILLOR ATTRITION ON POLITICAL PARTIES

We suggest that the relatively short lifespan of elected representatives, demonstrated above, will prove problematic for political parties that sponsor them. A proliferation of ward vacancies will presumably concern all political parties, particularly since it challenges them to spend more funds to bolster or sustain their portfolio in local government. Some political parties will cope better with attrition because of their size and potential to attract and develop new leaders, while others may be too fragile to absorb the shocks of increased AIDS deaths.

Chirambo (2008) argues that the party structures will be affected at three levels:
- leadership,
- finance, and
- administration/electioneering.

LEADERSHIP

Attrition due to AIDS or other causes among ward councillors may compromise the ability of small parties to regain their seats through by-elections, contributing to the dominance of a single party. Internally, unless there are clear succession plans and leadership pools to draw from, such parties may, over time, find themselves in decline as their most charismatic and experienced leaders succumb to diseases or AIDS-related complexes. This may impact on their effectiveness as an opposition party, their policy influence in local government and their appeal to the community at large.

FINANCE

South Africa has an institutionalised party financing system, which supports parliamentary political parties with funds proportionate to the seats they hold. In real terms, the larger parties would be better financed and prepared to compete in several by-elections at a time, while new parties may find it exceedingly difficult to sustain themselves. The chief electoral officer, in accordance with the Public Funding of Represented Political Parties Act of 1997, dispenses party funding. Funds are allocated according to a formula that takes into account the proportion of members a party has in the National Assembly and the provincial legislatures, and a minimum threshold amount to ensure equity. Private funding is not regulated (EISA: 2007).

Increased by-elections could still strain party finances, the municipal budget and the Independent Electoral Commission's (IEC's) resources, given the numbers and time involved.

Political parties will need to campaign for each by-election or series of by-elections that are called. Depending on how many vacancies occur due to death and other causes, the organisational, financial and electioneering capacity of political parties will be stretched.

ADMINISTRATION/ELECTIONEERING

Elections come with demands for advertising, community meetings, voter education and travel, among other commitments. The parties that have relatively well-organised and skilful administrators and campaigners are likely to prevail. In short, the death of a leader or several leaders should cause an entire political organisation's key structures, including its grassroots structures such as ward and branch committees, to swing into action to ensure a favourable outcome in all by-elections. The consequence is that, where parties fail to compete effectively, they will surrender space in council to the opposition.

NUMBER OF DECEASED COUNCILLORS PER PARTY

As we analyse the data, we should critically consider that the effects of councillor mortality transcend the boundaries of the local authority. They are also likely to affect the agencies that sponsor them: the political parties.

In this study, we note that, in absolute terms, the ANC experienced the most deaths among councillors at 202, which translates into 70,88% of all deaths; followed by the Inkatha Freedom Party (IFP) at 57 (20%), the Democratic Alliance at 18 (6,32%), and the New National Party (NNP) at 3 (1,05%). The United Democratic Movement (UDM) had the least deaths at 1 (0,35%) councillor. The deaths of four independent councillors constitute 1,40% of the total number of deaths recorded among ward representatives.

The number of councillors who are deceased amount to two-thirds of South Africa's national parliament of 400 members. On the face of it, the numbers can lead us to draw some misleading conclusions. While it is indeed evident that the ANC suffered the most in terms of absolute number of deaths, this may not be the case in relative terms. The 202 deceased councillors may represent a small fraction of the ANC's total number of representatives in local government, as it is the dominant party. Similarly, a party such as the UDM, which lost only one councillor, would have lost more in relative terms owing to its relatively smaller level of representation. However, purely in terms of the human and economic costs of replacing the deceased, these figures begin to gain more weight. Firstly, losing 202 people in six years among the leadership, whatever the cause of deaths, is not a phenomenon to be ignored.

Figure 10: Councillor mortality per political party (2001–2007)

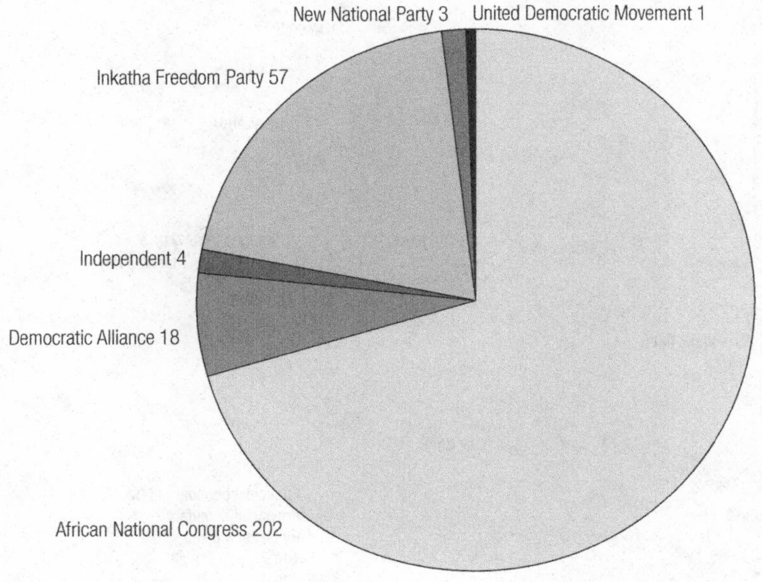

Source: IEC; calculations by Idasa.

The majority of the deaths occuring among councillors younger than 51 should raise the alarm over institutional memory and effective local governance. How can we possibly expect to build capacity in politics if the people who should lead will die before the age of 50? Coupled to this early mortality, if one considers that councillors view politics as a possible career choice, such high mortality among elected officialdom decreases the possible pool of skills and experience from which national politicians and parliamentary candidates can be drawn. This is likely to influence the type of candidates parties can field over time, with the net effect being weaker representation, skill erosion and political representation prone to ageing or subject to stagnation.

RELATING BY-ELECTIONS TO THEIR MUNICIPALITIES

As already suggested, the political party is only one institution that stands to feel the shocks of premature mortality among its leadership. Local authorities face the onerous task of dedicating time and resources to substituting the deceased through regular by-elections. It stands to reason that the municipal councils located in high HIV-prevalence areas will be more concerned about this, assuming HIV/AIDS is the cause of most vacancies.

Locating by-elections and deceased councillors in their respective municipalities has not been easy, given that municipal boundaries changed during 2001–2007. We therefore undertook to apportion the by-elections held in the old demarcations to the nearest new boundaries to appreciate how each institutional unit may be affected.

Figure 11: Elections per municipality (2001–2007)

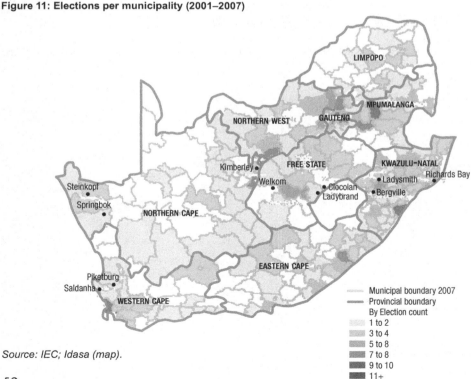

Source: IEC; Idasa (map).

The map shows that by-elections generated by various causes affected all municipalities. The numbers fluctuate from one province to the other. Municipalities located in Mpumalanga, Free State and KwaZulu-Natal held the most by-elections. The western half of the Northern Cape held the least, mainly due to its sparse population and its comparatively low level of HIV prevalence (Dorrington, et al.: 2006).

LOCATING BY-ELECTIONS CAUSED BY DEATH IN THEIR RESPECTIVE MUNICIPALITIES

The general picture does not tell us very much unless we can isolate the by-elections caused by death. Extrapolating the deaths to their respective municipalities unravels some new dynamics. Firstly, nearly all the municipalities with the highest numbers of absolute deaths are located in provinces with double-digit HIV prevalence during the period of study: KwaZulu-Natal (21,9%), Mpumalanga (23,1%), Free State (19,2%) and Gauteng (15,8%). The Western Cape, with a prevalence of 3,2%, is relatively less affected than the other provinces, inclusive of the Northern Cape, which has a prevalence of 9,0% (HRSC: 2005).[6]

Figure 12: By-elections caused by councillor mortality (2001–2007)

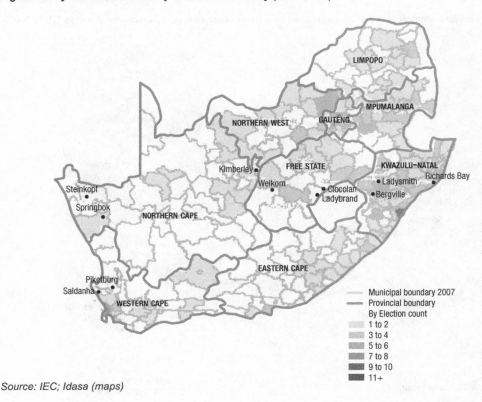

Source: IEC; Idasa (maps)

Municipalities in the Northern Cape experienced one or two deaths in the 2001–2007 period. The KwaZulu-Natal municipalities registered deaths ranging from seven to over 11 in the same period. Gauteng presents a similar pattern.

Among the 12 local municipalities sampled in this study, we find that KwaZulu-Natal local authorities experienced more deaths:

- Bergville, Ladysmith and Richards Bay all fall in the range of three to four by-elections resulting from the death of councillors.
- There were no by-elections caused by deaths in the Western Cape municipalities of Saldanha and Piketberg, although other areas of the province experienced upwards of 11 deaths during the 2001–2007 period.
- In the Northern Cape, of the four sampled municipalities, only Kimberley recorded one or two by-elections caused by the death of councillors.
- None of the five municipalities sampled in the Free State recorded any by-elections caused by the death of a councillor during this period. However, other municipalities, which did not form part of our sample, experienced between six and seven deaths among councillors between 2001 and 2007.

In relative terms, this picture may change. Figure 13 shows the by-elections caused by death as a percentage of total by-elections. In this analysis, we find that some of the municipalities with a low absolute number of deaths generate a higher percentage of deaths due the relatively smaller number of by-elections that occurred in general during this period.

Figure 13: Ward councillor mortality expressed as a percentage of total by-elections in wards (2001-2007)

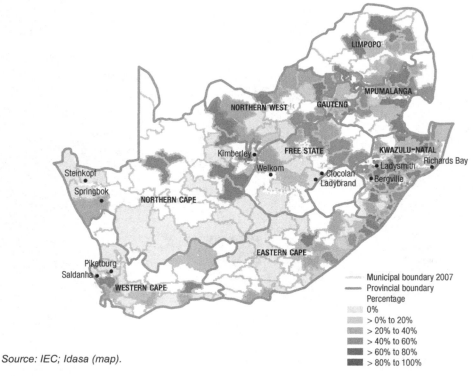

Source: IEC; Idasa (map).

In percentage terms, we find:

- In KwaZulu-Natal's Ladysmith and Bergville, 60–80% of all by-elections were caused by the death of a councillor. Richards Bay recorded 40–60% of vacancies arising due to the death of an elected local representative.
- There were no by-elections attributed to death in Saldanha and Piketberg in the Western Cape.
- In the Northern Cape, Kimberley saw 20–40% of its by-elections being caused by the death of a councillor.
- None of the five municipalities sampled in this study in the Free State experienced any by-elections resulting from death.

In both absolute and relative terms, the KwaZulu-Natal municipalities sampled in this study will have greater cause for concern regarding their mortality levels. These appear negligible if isolated within the municipalities sampled by Idasa. However, if we revert to the generic map (Figure 11), which shows the broader sample of local authorities across all nine provinces of South Africa, we might have a more compelling argument relating to the implications of by-elections in general and of death-induced by-elections in particular.

GOVERNANCE DYNAMIC: BY-ELECTIONS, POWER SHIFTS AND THE QUESTION OF ACCOUNTABILITY

In our analyses of the pattern of by-elections and their outcomes, we note that there are some shifts in representation in the local authority structures. We suggest that parties that fail to compete may lose policy influence as their numbers decline in the face of the epidemic. From the 589 by-elections held between 2001 and 2007, the major beneficiary has been the ANC. During the six years, the ANC won a total of 47 by-elections but lost 16, leaving its net gain at 31. The biggest losers have been the IFP with a net loss of –11, the UDM with –6, and the Democratic Alliance with –5. Some smaller parties, such as the Minority Front and the Independent Residence Party Association, had a net gain of 1, while the Freedom Front Plus had a net gain of 3. The New National Party had a net loss of –10. (This party was disbanded on 11 April 2005 and absorbed into the ANC.)

The information raises the possibility of a weakened opposition in the local government sector. Given the myriad issues associated with local government in South Africa, it may be logical to assume that the presence of a robust, energetic opposition is likely to raise the level of accountability as the party in power will constantly try to prove its worth through improved service delivery.

There are, therefore, three ways in which we suggest accountability may be affected:

- The accountability function of the opposition is weakened as AIDS deaths mount and parties fail to retain seats through subsequent by-elections.
- The dominant party becomes less accountable due to lowering threat perceptions.
- Conversely, the dominant party may be effective, wary of surrendering territory to the opposition in the foreseeable future.

In the first instance, opposition parties lose their influence in local government as their numbers dwindle. Minority parties are the most affected; therefore the voices of the marginalised become less pronounced or completely excluded. Enforceability of decisions is likely to be undermined, thereby undermining the principle of accountability over time.

In the second scenario, there may be a lack of responsiveness by members of the dominant party to the needs of their communities between elections due to the obvious reduced threat perception of a weakened opposition. The level of responsiveness might increase as elections draw closer, given that there would be a need to retain seats, but will go into a lull through most of their period in office. Answerability to the community may be the casualty here.

In the third scenario, and on a more positive note, a dominant party may seek to entrench itself and therefore pursue robust policies that uplift the welfare of the millions marginalised by poverty and disease.

LOSS OF REPRESENTATION AND THE QUESTION OF EFFECTIVE GOVERNMENT

There are other political costs associated with the death of a representative, which Idasa has documented in previous studies (Chirambo: 2008). These relate to the possible loss of representation for the community when their elected decision-maker dies.

The local government Municipal Structures Act of 1998 (Act 117 of 1998) Section 25(1)(d)(3)(d) states that a by-election must be held within 90 days of nomination day and that the MEC for local government must, after consultation with the IEC, determine the date of the election. During this period, important and urgent matters of service delivery may arise from among the electorate deserving immediate political attention.

In a country such as South Africa the level of civic awareness appears to be high. If the constant service-delivery protests are seen as an indicator, this might pose some tensions and even lead to violent clashes between citizens and authorities. However, there are indications from this study that the administrative system of local government in South Africa has been primed to shore up the deficits of the political system, depending on the nature of the issue. There are also various mechanisms that may be catalysed to fill the gap left by a deceased councillor:

- The speaker deals with the community on political matters in the absence of a councillor (deceased, expelled, etc.).
- The party that loses a councillor is allowed to appoint a temporary (PR) councillor, who may, in turn, appoint a coordinator for the ward.
- A liaison officer is appointed to address matters affecting the community that has lost a councillor.

The office of the speaker is responsible for matters dealing with community participation and, in well-resourced municipalities, will provide liaison officers to support ward councillors (Interview: Maujane). Matters that are channelled to the councillor from the electorate are analysed by the liaison officers. Should the matter be administrative in nature – for example, relating to the installation of a community water source – such a case would be directed to the responsible departments (Interview: Maujane). Should the matter be political, it will be channelled to the management of the municipality, which integrates it into the council agenda. The matter may be directed to the committee responsible for the respective area, which, in turn, advances its recommendations to the Executive Committee (EXCO). The EXCO will make its recommendation to the council, which then passes a decision on the matter (ibid.).

In the absence of a councillor, a liaison officer will undertake to engage the community on matters of concern and the communication process will, according to Maujane, continue uninterrupted. These linkages, however, will be dependent on the extent to which the speaker and mayor work together to enable a smooth process in the absence of a ward councillor.

The office of the speaker may organise for the mayor to address a community *Imbizo* to deal with a particularly pressing matter. This point is reinforced, among others, by the municipal managers of Beaufort West (Bhobhofolo), Okhahlamba and Nama Khoi municipalities.

Explaining this process, Beaufort West (Bhobhofolo) municipal manager said a PR councillor would be appointed by the speaker to fill the seat of a ward councillor should a vacancy occur due to death, resignation, expulsion or other causes. The speaker in this mayoral executive type council will handle the affairs of the community. His counterpart at Okhahlamba stated: '…the mayor, since he is a full-time councillor, he will be able to handle the community affairs'.

In the metros, some clear guidelines are followed. The Tshwane Metropolitan Municipality's by-law on ward committees, for example, states that when a ward councillor is no longer in office, the ward committee will continue to function for the rest of its term as determined by the council, and a temporary chairperson must be appointed by the political party that sponsored the original councillor. If the councillor was an independent candidate, the chief whip must appoint an interim chairperson from the PR councillors assigned to the ward. The new or interim councillor must re-appoint a coordinator for the ward (Tshwane ward committee by-laws: n.d.).

This study therefore finds that South Africa's local government system provides administrative mechanisms to deal with communities in the period when there is no representative (either due to death, resignation or expulsion). In this sense, we cannot assume that there is ineffectiveness. What we can question and further investigate is whether the established regulations and mechanisms are consistently applied – if at all – when there is a loss of representation.

We should be concerned, for instance, about the Auditor-General's 2006/2007 report, which raises alarm about the inability of municipalities to meet the needs of their communities. According to the report, 60% of the municipalities in South Africa cannot reconcile expenditure and receipts. The Auditor-General also draws a link between poor financial and administrative capacity and the current political instability in the country over lack of service delivery (*Mail & Guardian*: 26/06/08).

- Some 10% of municipalities did not submit financial statements to the Auditor-General, defying his order.
- Almost one-third of municipal funds are mismanaged and have been described as wasteful expenditure.

- More than 50% of municipalities could not account for the bulk of their expenditure and their financial statements are hence unreliable.
- The worst performers are listed as municipalities from Limpopo, Mpumalanga, North West, Northern Cape and Free State provinces.

(Politicsweb: 2008)

Given this revelation, we have to express grave doubts as to whether substitute councillors or liaison officers will be able to deliver effective government. In addition, would communities consider a PR councillor, a liaison officer or a ward coordinator a legitimate substitute for a directly elected ward councillor?

COST OF BY-ELECTIONS AND THE SUSTAINABILITY QUESTION

Thus far, this analysis has focused largely on human cost. We have assessed to some degree the impact of deaths among councillors, many of which may be related to AIDS, in the context of institutional capacity, accountability and effectiveness. Apart from the human cost, there are financial considerations to the local authorities of replacing deceased councillors and of filling vacancies that occur for a variety of reasons.

According to Michael Hendrickse, a senior officer at the IEC of South Africa, a ward by-election costs, on average, R25 000 (US$3 333) (Interview: Hendrickse). Based on this figure, South Africa spent at least R14,7 million (US$1,9 million) on hosting by-elections between 2001 and 2007.

At least half of that amount – R7,1 million (US$946 667) was spent in the wards where councillors died of undisclosed causes, compared to R6 million (US$800 000) to fill vacancies caused by resignations, R1 million (US$133 333) due to termination of services of councillors and R300 000 (US$40,000) for the dissolution of council. We note that deaths among councillors generate more costs to the Mixed Member Proportional (MMP) system than other causes. If we fall back on Dorrington, et al.'s report on AIDS deaths for 2004, we may add that 70% of all by-election costs related to death may be related to HIV/AIDS.

There is no indication at this point that any of the municipalities are in immediate danger of failing to sustain the wave of by-elections. Nor are there such indications from the IEC. Hendrickse, in fact, asserts that the IEC has adequate resources to sustain local by-elections; the costs are almost entirely covered by the IEC, except in cases where they may need specific support from the municipalities. However, there is sufficient alarm shown by municipal managers that these trends are worrisome from a financial perspective.

A municipal manager from Bergville underlined the significance of losing a ward councillor thus:

> It costs a lot, because you look at all the councillors that are involved. It is better
> if the councillors that passed on was a councillor from a political party that is in
> power and on top of that, the PR ... if it is a by-election it is costing a lot.
> (Municipal manager, Bergville)

Other respondents acknowledge the burden brought about by these special elections:

> *We budget for by-elections, so we budget R180 000 in case of emergency. [Each
> election costs] … in the region of R25 000. This is an estimated figure.*
> (IDP, Springbok)

A municipal manager in Kimberley said his council had experienced at least five by-elections in a five-year period:

> *Well, my rough estimate for such by-elections is something in the range of
> R70-80 000 … [by-elections in the last five years]… I think it is about five.*
> (Municipal manager, Kimberley)

OPPORTUNITY COSTS

While the IEC might, at this stage, not be strained financially by elections, we need to consider other related costs carried by political actors in these elections – particularly the political parties. The situation will favour parliamentary political parties that are awarded state funds based on their previous electoral performance. It does not bode well for the emergent political parties seeking to gain access to decision-making mechanisms in the interim. We need to reiterate, however, that even among the parliamentary parties, resources are distributed proportionate to the seats held in the National Assembly.

As noted earlier, political party funding is determined through the Public Funding of Represented Political Parties Act of 1997. Its provisions state that political parties shall be allocated public funds in proportion to the number of seats they hold in the National Assembly and provincial legislatures to reinforce the idea of proportionality in representation. From the allocation, 90% is paid at the start of the financial year. The remaining 10% becomes a provincial allocation. The funds are divided according to the seats in each provincial legislature, and each political party in each legislature takes an equal share of the allocation.

According to the Electoral Institute of Southern Africa (EISA) (2008), a party may use the funds for any purpose 'compatible with its functioning as a political party in a modern democracy'. Acceptable party uses of public funds include:
* campaigning,
* influencing public opinion,
* inspiring and furthering political education,
* promoting active citizen participation in political matters,
* influencing political trends, and
* promoting continuous links between the people and state structures.

The following are deemed unacceptable party uses of public funds:
* It is not permitted to give income to persons already in the employ of the state, in parliament, provincial legislatures or local authority.
* Party funds may not be used to finance causes or events that contravene the ethics by which Members of Parliament or any provincial legislature are bound.

- Party funds derived from public sources may not be used to establish any business, or acquire or maintain any right or financial interest whatsoever in any business or immovable property, unless it is for the sole and ordinary use of party-political purposes.
- Funds may not be used to undermine the functioning of a modern democracy.

A qualified auditor must audit all party funding from public sources. Each year, an income and expenditure statement of the year's funding must be prepared and submitted to the IEC for verification and auditing. Currently, there is no legislation prescribing the disclosure or monitoring of party funding from private donors and fund sources.[7]

Similarly, it could be assumed that some of the voters will be in gainful employment or involved in some form of economic activity. Their regular involvement in by-elections may reduce their contribution to the well-being of their communities.

VOTER PARTICIPATION AND THE QUESTION OF LEGITIMACY

The possible consequence of numerous by-elections is low participation from a public that is ridden with other survival priorities. Project Consolidate has already identified low participation in local government as a key challenge to municipalities and their legitimacy. It has been argued that democracies thrive on high participation as it increases the levels of legitimacy of the winner, given that the majority would have endorsed them (Strand & Chirambo: 2005). Relatively higher participation would also feed into the wider 'answerability' of a candidate to the electorate, who would view him or her as their product and commissioned to deliver on a number of their felt needs.

The premise here is that low participation is problematic for democracy. Voter mortality alone will not impact on legitimacy, but there are a number of related factors that can:

- Voter mortality may decrease the voter pool, impacting on participation rates.
- AIDS illness could constrain registered voters from voting (this was noted in previous studies by Idasa – see Strand & Chirambo: 2005).
- Care-giving could constrain participation due to contending priorities of survival (ibid.).
- Stigma and discrimination might also have similar effects, as noted in rural KwaZulu-Natal (ibid.).
- Repeated by-elections do have the tendency of attracting relatively fewer voters.

The question arises as to whether by-elections experience significantly lower participation rates than general elections or, in this case, local government elections. The absence of data from the IEC at the time of publishing this report constrains us from making these comparisons and, therefore, making any useful policy proposals in this section of the study.

However, some examples from the 12 municipalities studied show that of nine municipalities that held by-elections between 2001 and 2003, none achieved 50% participation. In effect, seven municipalities failed to reach 38% turnout, as indicated in Table 8.

Table 8: By-elections in selected municipalities (2001–2003)				
Municipalities	By-election date	Registered voters	Total votes cast	Percentage of poll
Sol Plaatjie	July 2001	4 529	1 450	32%
Masilonyana	October 2001	3 315	766	23,11%
Emnambithi-Ladysmith	November 2001	3 533	1 384	39,17%
uMhlathuze	May 2002	2 977	630	21,16%
Sol Plaatjie	June 2002	3 895	1 849	47,47%
Okhahlamba	July 2002	3 370	1 232	36,56%
Nama Khoi	August 2002	2 291	620	27,06%
Sol Plaatjie	November 2002	5 111	1 591	31,13%
Sol Plaatjie	May 2003	4 714	1 623	34,43%
uMhlathuze	May 2003	3 286	857	26,08%
Source: IEC website.				

VOTER ATTRITION AND RELATION TO
HIV/AIDS

Participation may also be complicated by increased mortality among voting age populations (VAPs) and registered voters. A depletion of the registered voter population might not seem significant when viewed from a national perspective. However, extrapolated to a provincial or municipal level, the impression may quite easily change.

If municipality X is located in a high-HIV prevalence area, it is likely to register more deaths among its community and, therefore, its voters over time. Such an impact may be felt through an increase in the demand for cemetery space and consistently lower attendance at the local polls. Municipality X would therefore have a greater need to raise more concerns about its community than municipality Y, which has a single-digit prevalence rate.

This hypothetical scenario, however, only holds if we assume that all registered voters remained in the provinces or localities where they registered for the last six years or so.

We know, of course, that South Africa experiences several forms of human mobility, including rural-urban migration (IOM [PHAMSA]: 2005).

This implies that, while the voters may register in one area, they will not necessarily die there. Increased deaths among the registered and voting-age population also has the added potential of causing authorities to reconsider constituency boundaries. Constituencies are demarcated with more or less similar size populations.

Because AIDS disproportionately affects 14–49 year olds, it may skew the size of constituency populations, rendering some wards much smaller population-wise (Chirambo: 2008). Delimitation exercises are costly and will challenge the government to set aside additional resources for the process.

The third and last level of impact on participation would be political party involvement. While it is not within the scope of this study to establish party memberships, it

61

is worth mentioning that political parties that draw membership primarily from younger members of the community will be most affected by the loss of this demographic.

VOTER MORTALITY (1999–2006)

Data released in 2007 by the IEC indicates that 2 679 713 registered voters died between 1999 and 2006. This means that South Africa loses, on average, 27 914 registered voters on a monthly basis.

The data also shows that the 30–39 and 40–49 age groups are the two most affected age cohorts. Deaths among 30–39 year olds rose steadily between 1999 and 2002, and peaked in 2004 before stabilising marginally in 2005 and 2006. More than 90 000 individuals in this age cohort died prematurely (before age 40).

Figure 14: Voter mortality (1999–2006)

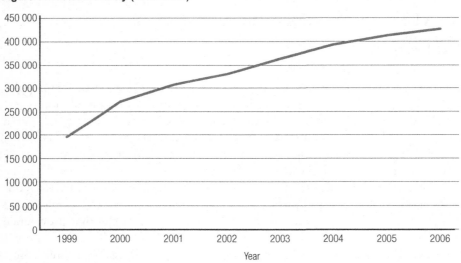

Source: IEC; calculations by Idasa.

The 40–49 age cohort experienced a few dips between 2000 and 2002, but peaked around 2004 and continued on an upward trend. Casualties translated into 80 000 in terms of absolute numbers of deaths. These trends are less evident in 20–29 year olds.

The trends in deaths among male and female voters, when aggregated, exhibit the same upward spiral since 1999, with only marginal stability between 2002 and 2004.

More than 200 000 of each gender died during the 1999–2006 period, with the number of female deaths slightly higher than that of males.

Figure 15: Voter mortality by age cohort (1999–2006)

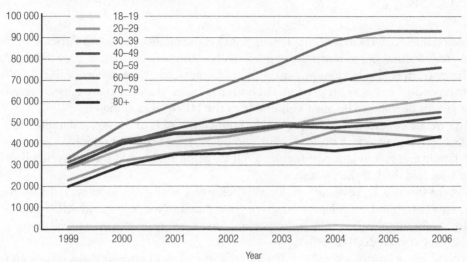

Source: IEC; calculations by Idasa.

Figure 16: Voter mortality by gender (1999–2006)

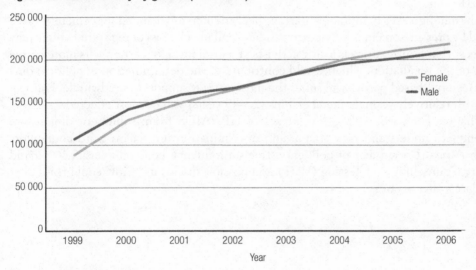

Source: IEC; calculations by Idasa.

The experience of increased deaths among poor South Africans of a voting age may be attributable to an irregular health system inclined towards servicing upper-middle and upper class societies with higher quality care. While the public health sector is large and offers free services subsidised by the state, it does not compete in quality with the rapidly expanding private sector, which boasts highly specialised hi-tech health services. Middle- and high-income earners, usually supported by medical aid schemes, largely use the private health care system (Meritor Consulting, 2005).

CONCLUSION

The discussion and analyses in this chapter suggest that the majority of South Africa's ward councillors are succumbing to mortality at a relatively young age (i.e. before they reach 50 years). This pattern is also evident among registered voters, where members of the 30–49 age cohort have died in larger proportions. In both instances, the deaths are concentrated in the age groups deemed to be most vulnerable to the HIV/AIDS epidemic.

The experience of personal loss expressed by councillors adds to the general impression that AIDS is having an effect on leadership. Some 59,4% of the respondents said they had lost a family member, relation or friend to AIDS; while 16,8% said they knew a fellow councillor who had died of the disease.

The loss of elected representatives for this relatively young democracy, is likely to under-cut efforts to build capacity for effective government. Not only could AIDS illness play a part in absenteeisms, it may be responsible for some resignations as well (which stood at 40,9% between 2001-2006).

The second important observation relates to the similarities between these trends and the AIDS mortality profile described by Dorrington, et al. (2006) and UNAIDS/WHO (2006). In both instances, we note that South Africa's average life expectancy is calculated at 51 years.

Deaths among VAPs in municipalities are likely to increase demand for cemetery space preceded by pressure on clinic services as residents fall ill. The loss of registered voters may also suggest that South Africa is losing activists at a local level, or certainly its more active segment of the population, which would contribute to the determination of political outcomes. Regional-based parties will suffer the most as their support bases dwindle. Political parties with relatively younger memberships (20–49 years) will be most affected.

In Chapter Four, we explore the impact of HIV/AIDS from a different dimension. We attempt to understand how stigma and discrimination impact on ward councillors in South Africa. Does a fear of political ostracism influence political decisions to avoid Voluntary Counselling and Testing (VCT) and possibly disclosure? How could this affect a candidate's effectiveness?

CHAPTER FOUR

THE IMPACT OF STIGMA AND DISCRIMINATION ON WARD COUNCILLORS

The objective of this chapter is to understand in what ways stigma and discrimination affect elected local officials who may be HIV-positive. Could being HIV-positive cause an elected official to withdraw from public functions and responsibilities from time to time? If so, how would this affect their effectiveness and accountability to the communities who, by law, must be engaged every quarter by their representatives on a range of needs? What are the underlying causes of fear of Voluntary Counselling and Testing (VCT) and disclosure among councillors?

We learn from mortality statistics that death is responsible for 48,7% of vacancies in the political establishment at local level (see Chapter Three). It was also noted that the majority of councillors died before the age of 51. The mortality profile was closely related to the HIV/AIDS trends we have become accustomed to over the last 25 years, where 15–49 year olds have been most affected.

There is, in addition, a fairly strong impression described by councillors of their personal experience of loss to HIV/AIDS: 59,4% of the respondents indicated they had lost a family member, relation or friend to AIDS, while 16,8% said they knew a fellow councillor/s who had died of the epidemic.

The chapter is therefore foregrounded by the understanding that councillors face similar experiences of HIV/AIDS as the communities they serve. It stands to reason therefore to assume that the stigma and discrimination experienced by ordinary folk might also be extended to elected officials who exhibit symptoms of illness or are openly living with HIV. In this regard, we interviewed 112 councillors in the 12 municipalities on their experience of HIV/AIDS, strategic interaction with the epidemic and their communities, and the potential impact of stigma and discrimination on their careers. To illustrate a complete picture of how the epidemic might possibly generate these phenomena, we also spoke to municipal manger, Integrated Development Plan (IDP) managers and HIV/AIDS officers within those councils.

The respondents were asked questions in the following thematic areas:
- disclosure
- careers (real and perceived effect), and
- policies (proposals by councillors to deal with stigma).

This discussion is motivated by the findings presented by Idasa (Chirambo: 2008), which suggest that politicians who are HIV-positive may be marginalised from aspiring to political office by their political parties, or live in constant fear of rejection by their parties and the electorate.

DEFINING STIGMA AND THE SCOPE OF INTERROGATION

Ogden & Nyblade (2005) cite an established UNICEF definition developed by Goffman in the 1960s, which describes stigma as a systematic 'process of devaluation' brought about by a pervasive negative association connected to a person, practice or event. In the context of HIV/AIDS, stigmatisation is a by-product of deeper stigmatisations attached to behaviour, moral codes, gender, race, religion, class and negative interpretations of other forms of social membership by a dominant social mindset. These stigmatisations frequently involve inaccurate or inappropriate value judgements attached to the behaviours associated with HIV/AIDS transmission and infection, and those unfortunate enough to be infected by it. In this, HIV/AIDS is often associated with sexual promiscuity, immorality, intravenous drug usage and rebellion against authority.

In the perpetrator-victim duality of stigmatisation, we can extend the definition of stigma by partitioning it into two categories: 'felt' stigma and 'enacted' stigma. Felt stigma refers to the perception of public judgement one expects to experience if one is associated with the negative behaviours that draw on stigmatising beliefs. Enacted stigma is directly related to the actual discriminatory practices to which the individual is subject (Mnyanda: 2006). The process of devaluation, it appears, is dualistic in nature and emerges from how one expects to be treated and how one is treated.

Stigma is both contingent on human perceptions of others and the environments in which these perceptions are formed. Goffman identifies three types of physical and psychological associations that give rise to stigmas and discriminations. The first relates to disfigurements or abominations of the body; the second to deficiencies or perversions in character; and the third to generic negative profiles of other communities, nations or races.

All three types of discriminations strive to create an exclusion or otherness based on perceptions of 'us' and 'them' (Ogden & Nyblade: 2005; Mfecane & Skinner: 2004).

In the creation of negative perceptions, Parker & Aggleton (2003) suggest that the 'us' and 'them' attached to HIV stigmatisation can influence the way in which social power relationships and memberships are formed. These resultant skewed power relationships have the effect of replicating inequalities in social status and membership. Ogden & Nyblade (2005) reiterate Parker and Aggleton's point that social sectoral solidarity, created by the imposition of a label or otherness upon members of society, deepens and sharpens existing social inequalities attached to social membership, leading to discrimination.

In this sense, stigma assigns roles and values to people that are not really theirs, and the stigmatised label becomes a means of controlling who is permitted to participate in society and who is not. Determining the source of devaluation and discrediting of persons emerges from our deeper understandings of political participation within institutions and communities.

It is simplistic to say that a medical condition alone results in stigmatisation, unless that condition is associated with something else considered more insidious. In the context of HIV and the stigma it attracts, behaviours and moral codes, or lack thereof, are associated with the acquisition of the virus. Such behaviours are usually linked to sexual promiscuity, sexual deviance and intravenous drug usage (Mfecane & Skinner: 2004; Ogden & Nyblade: 2005; Mnyanda: 2006).

This constitutes the basis for the formation of 'us' and 'them' labels, and will in all probability influence the extent and scope of social participation the stigmatised or persons fearing stigmatisation will experience.

CONTEXTUALISING STIGMA AND DISCRIMINATION IN SOUTH AFRICA

What makes stigma particularly dangerous in South African social and political terms is that it tends to drive the discourse on HIV/AIDS underground, thereby minimising the chances that behaviour and attitudes will change. The stigma associated with HIV infection, and the broader social unwillingness to discuss it, disrupts the functioning of society and its institutions by introducing 'a desire not to know one's own status, thus delaying testing and accessing treatment' (Mfecane & Skinner: 2004). The generic stigmatisation of People Living With HIV and AIDS (PLWHAs) is indicative of a discriminatory regimen that cannot address contentious issues in the open, which has the tendency to hamper prevention and awareness campaigns and hamper containment initiatives.

Behaviours have been slow to modify as people have demonstrated a noted unwillingness to admit that the disease exists. Denial on a massive social scale prevents effective steps from being taken to reduce HIV/AIDS prevalence. So deep is the stigma that people have been known to refuse testing and treatment – the core means of addressing awareness and containment programmes. Mfecane & Skinner (2004) have suggested in their three-year study that even preventative measures are seen as associative of infection, so anyone who practises preventative measures is stigmatised as being a possible HIV carrier. The use of condoms, for example, signifies the spread of the epidemic, and anyone initiating their usage is automatically labelled or rejected. Certain conceptions of masculinity can also lead to stigmatisation and social marginalisation. In some parts of society, monogamous relationships are derided where polygamy or many concurrent relationships are viewed as proof of manhood.

The immediate threat HIV poses to the individual is lessened by an act of 'distancing'. In other words, HIV, like syphilis, is viewed as the disease of the 'deviant' and the 'immoral', and therefore of little concern to those who hold socially respectable beliefs about masculinity or femininity. Beliefs informing personal behaviour are seldom self-scrutinised. This view results in the portrayal of women as the carriers and dominant transmitters of HIV. Such views further undermine broader social attempts to attain inclusive social and political practises (Mfecane & Skinner: 2004).

HIV, STIGMA AND EXCLUSION

Common general perceptions of sexual excess and moral deviancy fuel the views underpinning HIV stigmatisation (Shefer: 2004; Mfecane & Skinner: 2004). These perceptions frame HIV in notions of fear and retribution. In some communities, the fear of HIV is so deeply entrenched that those living with HIV are ostracised, and sometimes even killed.

Within the context of how stigma is defined, felt stigma is reinforced by genuine discriminatory behaviour. The mob murder of Gugu Dlamini, an HIV activist who openly declared her status is an extreme example. Another woman was raped and later murdered after her attackers discovered that she was HIV-positive. Other forms have manifested in the exclusion of HIV-positive children from attending crèche or school. Discrimination in the workplace has been the most common. All these experiences appear to demonstrate deeply ingrained forms of stigma and discrimination in South African society (Chirambo: 2008; Mfecane & Skinner: 2004).

STIGMA IN POLITICS

Broader social stigmatisation related to HIV seems very likely to manifest in political arrangements, particularly at the local level where these prejudicial beliefs may be held by larger proportions of people who are less informed about HIV/AIDS. It seems plausible, given the pervasiveness of discrimination against people living with HIV, that councillors and politicians in general will be socially stigmatised by the messages they send out to communities, and by the information they choose to publicly disclose.

What emerges is a complex position that cannot be covered by a few general statements. Our aim is not to unpack this complexity, but to provide some indication of the difficulty attached to public office in dealing with stigma and negative associations emerging from institutional and community sources.

In this, stigma is directly derivative of the denial of PLWHA's participation in decision-making.[8] Additionally, in the absence of HIV-positive people in leadership roles, and the possible reluctance of existing leadership to engage with the issue, it would be necessary for lobby groups and the infected themselves to identify friendly faces within current political leadership to initiate policies that represent the interests and cater to the needs of the infected (Chirambo: 2008).

FINDINGS

DISCLOSURE

Political leaders fear rejection, but anyone can get it. (Councillor, Piketberg)

There is a fear of ostracism among councillors that influences their attitudes toward disclosure, VCT and Anti-retroviral Therapy (ART). Except for one female councillor in the Free State, none of the respondents disclosed HIV-positive statuses. The dominant opinion suggests that HIV-positivity is anathema among their communities and may result in councillors losing their support bases or careers.

These views resonate with previous findings, where some HIV-positive rural voters in KwaZulu-Natal withdrew from the electoral process due to a fear of discrimination and violent attacks from other members of the community (Strand & Chirambo: 2005). It reinforces findings on discrimination by the Department of Health conducted in 2002, which indicated high levels of stigma and discriminatory attitudes in South Africa against PLWHAs (Jennings et al: 2002).

While there is no basis for us to suggest that these levels of discrimination have since remained constant, we can at least interrogate how a leadership in denial might negatively affect any measure of progress gained against stigma and discrimination in the past four years

In this ASCI study, we note that councillors were happy to disclose the event of their testing only where the results proved negative. An HIV coordinator from Richards Bay, for instance, underscored this observation, which materialised from discussions with respondents. In the coordinator's opinion, more benefit would come from politicians disclosing their HIV-positive status to challenge the assumptions of HIV being a disease of the poor, the uneducated, the immoral and the sexually promiscuous.

> It is kept a secret, so we do not really know who has died from AIDS.
> (Councillor, Steinkopf)

The responses from the majority of councillors on disclosure contrast with the generally held view that the introduction of confidentiality and the availability of ART will lead to increased openness and public testing. The views expressed by politicians in this study project an image of leaders who are as ordinary as the people they serve in terms of their hopes and fears about HIV/AIDS.

One councillor from Richards Bay remarked, '[E]ven now I can't go and test, not because I am a political leader. I was talking to my colleagues last month. I said I want to go and have myself tested but I didn't have the strength I needed.'

> I think what makes it difficult for any ordinary person would make it difficult for a political leader. The fact there is no cure for this disease and eventual death; it would be the same thing for a political leader himself, whether he can accept the fact that he is going to be dying because there is no cure for this disease.
> (HIV coordinator, Richards Bay)

> I sat with someone who was going to get tested. She was scared and that worry makes you ill. I told her she must go just for her own peace of mind … Only with my permission can another person release my status … (Councillor, Steinkopf)

The majority of opinions seem to suggest that reconciling their fears of testing and disclosure with their roles as leaders in their communities is a challenge for councillors. However, on a positive note, a minority view leaned towards greater openness as a way of raising awareness and showing leadership to communities. One councillor in Kimberley, echoing this minority position, expressed a belief that testing should be made mandatory due to a constitutional right to life.

DIVERSE VIEWS ON TESTING AND DISCLOSURE

> I was the first one to give the example by taking the test. (Councillor, Kimberley)

> People shy away from these testing sessions. They will not speak about it all that

easily and they are not comfortable with it … we have to cultivate this awareness.
We must keep at it and encourage people to talk about it.
(IDP manager, Springbok)

It is only when people are close to death when they discover they have got AIDS,
so there is a relative degree of secrecy. (District municipal manager, Springbok)

I think it is good if you disclose early, because the doors are open to you to get
treatment. A lot of people sometimes get sick because they cannot get proper treat-
ment. The people who suffer most are those who hide and disclose late.
(Councillor, Bergville)

We also noted that the willingness to disclose and support for testing can be located within the district and provincial prevalence rates. In the Northern Cape, where HIV prevalence is cited as relatively low, more councillors were less willing to disclose or suggest disclosure as a strategy for containing the social spread and escalating political costs of HIV/AIDS. Among councillors in KwaZulu-Natal, the province hardest hit by the AIDS epidemic, and councillors around the mines in the Free State, disclosure was seen as one of the most viable containment tools.

Given that councillors are viewed as agents of delivery, stigma and discriminatory practises can be active determinants in defining their participation in their communities and the execution of their community-determined delivery mandates. Disclosure can be a double-edged sword as discrimination is likely to strike from both sides of the institutional divide. One of the side effects of stigma is that people, including politicians, are more likely to be excluded on the basis of appearance. A cursory visual AIDS test is enough to exclude or stigmatise people who look ill or exhibit the symptoms associative of AIDS, such as rashes, sores and weight loss. Should a councillor exhibit these symptoms, our concern is that they could be excluded, or socially and politically marginalised, simply on the basis of their real or perceived medical status.

We cannot discount the idea that politicians in South Africa themselves may be discriminatory towards HIV sufferers – a possibility raised by a councillor from Welkom who observed that, 'They [the politicians] say you must not discriminate, but they are the people who discriminate. They will say, "Go and sit down because you are sick". They are the ones who discriminate but the policy is written by them.'

It is possible that the stigma is glossed over among politicians as the fears of the community may be present among councillors. One councillor in Ladybrand suggested the origin of ostracism in politics and in communities resides in a broader fear that can simply be based on a perception of HIV infection: '[P]eople will be afraid of him. They will be afraid and say that he is sick.' The fear among councillors is dual in that HIV status is perceived as a social ill and a political risk. This could further drive the stigma, and force discourses addressing this, underground. Evidence for these negative assumptions is gleaned from councillors and it is worth citing some of these opinions for illustrative value:

They can say terrible things about people, accuse you of sleeping around and
make insinuations around it. (Councillor, Springbok)

I think it is an embarrassment because people see it [HIV] as a dirty disease.
(HIV officer, Richards Bay)

[It is] the same as saying I am gay. The people will stone you; doesn't matter how you got it. Some people will understand that you can get it without doing immoral things, but most people will crucify you anyway. (Councillor, Ladybrand)

People are not open with their status. They tend to say that [an HIV-related] death is attributable to cancer. (IDP manager, Springbok)

What I have realised is that people will think that HIV is only for the people who are careless … (HIV-positive councillor)[9]

… people are in denial, they are not easily accepting … (Councillor, Warrenton)

The problem is that they are leading the community and are afraid to disclose … because some of the people will think that everyone in the party is sick.
(Councillor, Ladybrand)

EFFECTS OF HIV/AIDS ON POLITICAL CAREERS

The quote from the Ladybrand councillor on political perceptions of HIV is of tremendous value as it speaks to the need for ward councillors and political parties to politically address the stigma of HIV/AIDS. The impression created here is that, if members of a political party disclose, it can generate negative public perceptions of their organisation and possibly reduce it to ridicule in the eyes of its opponents. Parties may decide that the political costs of disclosure are too high and may conclude that it is not collectively worthwhile to address HIV's effect on the party.

This may inhibit the fielding of HIV-positive candidates and further marginalise an already stigmatised grouping. One councillor from Ladysmith remarked, in the context of disclosure, '… communities lose hope if they see politicians dying of AIDS.' Although a decidedly minority view, it is a significant view given the perceived sense of discrimination in society across South Africa.

One councillor from Clocolan expressed this sentiment well: 'I think they might start losing their support base. You see, if they lose their support, they might not be re-elected and people may say that that they don't want him or her anymore as a leader.'

For some councillors, the fear of marginalisation may go beyond their mandate and be personal in nature. A natural fear of losing one's job as a councillor could force them to publicly side with the dominant community voice, which could entrench discriminatory attitudes and the lack of willingness to disclose. One councillor, for example, observed that it is akin to a fear of losing everything one has.

I think today's people, if they know your status, they will not receive votes. I think they hide their status for reasons such as these. (Councillor, Clocolan)

*You will receive the vote if you say 'I have HIV'. You will receive the votes because
I saw with one of our practitioners who disclosed their status. The people were so
encouraged. They wished our leaders could do the same.*
(Councillor, Clocolan)

I don't think it [HIV] can affect anybody's political career.
(Councillor, Richards Bay)

The two contending views emerging from some municipalities regard the disclosure of a local politician with HIV/AIDS as being either political suicide or an inspirational force that may not only establish empathy with PLWHAs, but also catalyse openness among communities.

One councillor in Welkom stated that it could only bode well for a politician's career if he or she disclosed his or her status to the constituency. In the same municipal area, however, many diverse reasons were offered to support non-disclosure.

One councillor, echoing this stream of views, suggested, 'If I go for a public HIV test and you disclose your status and we go for elections in 2009, can you imagine what the opposition will do? ... So I will rather keep it to myself and my family.'

Socially, one councillor remarked, '[I]f I can tell you that I am HIV-positive, you are going to look at me like I am dirty.' Another councillor suggested that, 'AIDS in this country is still regarded as leprosy.'

The advent of ART notwithstanding, another councillor remarked that careers would suffer because, 'they are going to die before they can deliver what they are supposed to deliver in the community'. The unwillingness of councillors to disclose their status publicly is underpinned by a form of cynical fatalism and a lack of hope by those who, technically, in the opinion of many, should be a major part of the solution.

Councillors seem to worry more about what their voters may think than fundamentally how their political parties could react. Although the two concerns are interrelated, the impression constructed through this interview process suggested that local communities are not literate enough on matters of HIV/AIDS to accept a leader living openly with the virus.

*... [I]f people disclose their status, they think that it will negatively affect their
career because there is this misconception that this guy is going to die soon, so then
people will start to think that they don't need to vote him in because he can't finish
his term.* (Councillor, Free State)

LEADERSHIP: THE EXPERIENCE OF AN HIV-POSITIVE COUNCILLOR

These opinions are challenged by the compelling story of an HIV-positive councillor in the Free State, who lives openly with the condition and has not reported any harassment or exclusion from colleagues or political parties.

She is currently serving her second term in office and has had nothing but support from her colleagues. In an environment where denial appears rife, this novel case perhaps provides a first insight into how disclosure might affect a political leader. From her own account, she experiences no ostracism and is able to discharge her duties without hindrance. She has, however, implied experience of some form of socio-political barrier within her community, particularly when people have questioned why her party chose to adopt 'someone who is dying'. Her full remarks are recorded below.

> You should not let the virus rule your lifestyle because, in the end, how are you going to encourage others ... Some will come to me and say, 'How can the [name of political party omitted] send somebody who is busy dying?' And I will say, 'You know the [name of political party omitted] sent somebody who is busy dying because at least that person will be making a difference.' My colleagues have all along been very supportive, even in my first term of office, even in my second term ... My boss would call me and ask my opinion on certain things. Other councillors call me and say I need you to speak to this friend of mine. So that is how we interact. They know I can speak to people. I am openly living with HIV so they are making use of my services.

While the majority of councillors in this study seem to favour non-disclosure, there is a fairly respectable current of thought that shores up the case of the Free State councillor with regard to the leadership importance of openness.

THE INFLUENCE OF HIV ON A CAREER

> I strongly believe it [HIV disclosure] will affect it [career] positively. The people who come out and disclose their status are not taken lightly. They are taken as reliable people, as honest people; people who are prepared to lose.
> (Councillor, Theunissen)

> When you are a political leader, you are leading people. And by telling people your status, it is going to encourage many people. (Councillor, Ladybrand)

As one councillor remarked, 'I see absolutely nothing wrong because an HIV-positive person can stand a five-year chance. I have seen some get sick, but some have recovered. Some have served a five-year term, some are still in and some are out, so I do not see any problem.'

Others say that careers should suffer no ill effect and, if anything, should have a positive and encouraging effect on voters. A councillor for Theunissen offered this view: 'It is not going to affect it. It will encourage people because, when you are a political leader, you are leading people and by telling your status it is going to encourage many people.'

Another councillor indicated that disclosure could only increase the popularity of a candidate. It seems, therefore, albeit a minority view, that the disclosure of status to the wider electorate may have some positive effects.

EDUCATION AND POLICY FOR MANAGING STIGMA AND DISCRIMINATION

The lack of guidance from central government and the lack of visible policy implementation was enough to stimulate some councillors into claiming nothing was being done, or that not enough was being done, to prevent the spread of HIV or provide treatment to the infected.

Councillors cited education as one of the preventative strategies. Councillors themselves have raised considerable concerns about their own levels of education on HIV matters. One councillor from the Free State remarked, '[W]e need to be educated around it [HIV] as councillors and even in our homes. They must bring people who are well-trained and have the programme, so that they can come and educate us, make sure that the stigma is being taken away from us.' Education is, however, according to Mfecane & Skinner (2004), no comfortable panacea upon which we should pin our hopes of HIV containment, treatment and prevention.

If we were to open up a public discourse at the local level on HIV, as one councillor recommends, knowledge would indeed be an important element of prevention and policy initiatives, but by no means the only remedy.

To start the discussion, community leaders would have to be informed and acknowledge the importance of the need to recognise the extent of the issue. As one councillor eloquently said, '[E]very time you address the public, talk about it. It should actually be at the top of your agenda. AIDS is a part of us; we need to deal with it.'

On the part of individuals, knowledge of one's status, defined through testing, is cited as one of the core components of any prevention campaign and forms the basis of policy responses at the local level. A number of councillors expressed different opinions on the role and use of testing, but they all agreed that testing is a strategy worth considering in addressing the fears, stigmas and roles of social role models.

TESTING AS PART OF A WIDER SOLUTION

> If it is someone who is working [who is infected with HIV], we say this person is working and has the strength to work. So if you test, it does not mean that you are going to lose your job or your health, but you must know your status.
> (Councillor, Bergville)

> It [testing] has to be compulsory. Everybody must come out and be tested.
> (Councillor, Richards Bay)

> As politicians, we have to lead by example … we should go and test, and we should also try to talk to communities. (Councillor, Kimberley)

Fear and uncertainty, as drivers of stigma, have to be addressed in a public way. A councillor from Springbok stated that the only way we can deal with the disease is if HIV-positive people publicly disclose their status and then go on the road to tell people about how they were infected and how they are now living with the disease. This sentiment was mirrored in a view from a councillor from Theunissen: '[T]he whole question of treatment can be dealt with quite easily if a number of people declare openly, but speak positively about their own behaviour.'

To build on the issue of fear and whose issue stigma really is, one councillor stated that the solution resides in the collective ownership of the disease. Everyone must live as though they were infected with HIV. This would then require that we change our life-styles, eat healthily and conduct ourselves with care in our sexual relations.

> We have to take AIDS as something that is not choosy. It will go to anyone, even
> a minister, so we don't need to class it as a status thing … you can control it if you
> have information around it and take proper measures to protect yourself, but as
> for being embarrassed about having this disease, it is not going to have a negative
> impact on you or your community, so people must be taught that it is everyone's
> sickness. (Councillor, Theunissen)

One of the councillors raised the issue that ART supplies are irregular at their local clinic and that this would entail better management from the branches of government responsible for this. Proponents of the ART argument in this study see treatment as one of the weapons against stigma. Seeing a sick person recover challenges the assumption that HIV is equivalent to instant death. They also hold that senior government agents and politicians are part of the solution and should disclose their status. This would challenge the assumption that HIV/AIDS is a disease of the poor. Evidently, poverty is also highly stigmatised and part of the environment of HIV stigma.

Another cause for concern is the lack of information surrounding HIV infection levels in communities. Councillors have suggested that the lack of prevalence data at the local level makes it difficult to plan local responses and awareness campaigns.

CONCLUSION

Stigma is fed by assumptions of how HIV is transmitted. Certain expressions of sexuality and the intravenous usage of narcotics – the dominant means of HIV/AIDS transmission – attract a stigma that feeds the prejudice against those suffering from the disease, whether they display any of the 'deviancies' associated with the assumed behaviours or not. Such a prior association attracts discrimination that creates a differentiated form of treatment usually dismissive of the contributions and needs of the infected. Because of this, local politicians may be marginalised by their parties and by their colleagues, although further evidence for this would have to be gathered and determined from a separate study.

In one case, an HIV-positive councillor is openly living with HIV and receives support from her colleagues. Hers is an isolated case as many councillors did not disclose or speak freely on this issue, although some offered opinions on how we should deal with people living with HIV.

One of the core issues is that personal culpability is seen as the domain of the infected person alone. The stigma accompanying HIV infection does not make distinctions between the modes of infection. Some councillors described the social stigma attached to HIV as originating from promiscuous sexual behaviour and, therefore, that an HIV-positive person is 'dirty'. This leads to a broader social rejection of the person. Should local politicians disclose, they may be forced to resign or absent themselves from duty on a regular basis, fuelling ineffectiveness.

Other councillors questioned about the impact of HIV/AIDS did not believe that stigma was career ending, but many certainly held the view that it could be used to undermine their public credibility. Some even ventured that the opposition would lead the attack on the viability of elected representatives who openly declared their HIV status, although none admitted that they thought of their party colleagues as being a genuine source of political exclusion.

The majority of councillors expressed the need for education on HIV to reduce the stigma and silence surrounding HIV/AIDS. The absence of disclosure and the lack of knowledge, coupled with high infection rates in some communities, could deplete the pool from which future councillors may be drawn as people die in denial. This may introduce elements of fragility as councillors pass away and communities cannot field skilled, experienced and tested candidates for those positions.

Overall, the issues raised in this section challenge the traditional notion of leadership regarding HIV/AIDS. If leadership, in part, implies the ability to boldly respond to VCT, then it is clear that HIV-related stigma is compromising it. Unless approaches are devised to deal with this 'political stigma' we cannot expect public confidence in leaders to be sustained over time as evidence of hypocrisy surfaces.

Consequently, we could assume that a leadership in denial will be ineffective in governing the epidemic in the face of public mistrust about their sincerity and openness on HIV/AIDS.

CHAPTER FIVE

COMMUNITY PERSPECTIVES ON HIV/ AIDS AND THE ROLE OF COUNCILLORS

The notion of effectiveness and accountability, or the lack of it, was discussed at length in Chapter Four, particularly relating to how AIDS sickness may cause self-exclusion from public affairs among councillors. In this chapter, we examine how this might be compounded by the further possibility of ostracism of infected leaders by communities averse to People Living With HIV and AIDS (PLWHAs).

The thrust of this expanded discourse, therefore, is to understand better the challenges elected representatives are likely to face as they seek to perform their responsibilities on behalf of their communities. More specifically, the chapter also seeks to understand whether HIV-positive councillors might face impediments within their communities due to discrimination.

In relation to this, we ask: In an environment where concerns for improved welfare permeate society, would it really matter that an 'agent of change' carries a potentially life-threatening virus and is open about it? Would it matter less if the work is done? In general, what do people expect of their elected representatives in terms of service delivery on HIV/AIDS?

Afrobarometer studies give us a compelling picture of which sections of South African society are the most expectant of change in their social and economic circumstances, and how these expectations translate into public expressions of discontent when services are not seen to be delivered.

Historically disadvantaged people, in this case the black population of South Africa, have expressed more dissatisfaction with local service delivery than citizens in higher income brackets (Bratton & Sibanyoni: 2006). In our analysis of councillors' responses to a wide range of questions on their personal experience of HIV/AIDS, we infer a sense of apprehension about disclosing HIV statuses when one is a serving politician. Although there is a mixed reaction on whether openness on AIDS is helpful or not in the long run, we find only a single councillor who lives openly with HIV. We also understand that councillors are not particularly well equipped in terms of knowledge and strategies to deal with AIDS in their communities.

How, then, does this balance out against the expectations of their constituencies? How do ordinary rural folk perceive the roles of councillors and their impact on matters relating to the epidemic and service delivery? How would communities respond to a councillor who lives openly with HIV?

FOCUS GROUPS

To address these questions, we organised focus-group discussions (FGDs) with local residents. The rationale was to aim for depth rather than quantity in understanding citizen sentiments on their councillors' performance on HIV/AIDS matters. However, we need to add caution to these statements, given that the focus groups present opinions of a small sample, the results of which may not have external validity. There were eight focus groups in the four provinces studied. Respondents were selected from their communities and factors such as HIV status, gender, age, level of political participation and employment status were taken into account. The urban or rural origin of the participants was also considered. FGDs were conducted in English, Afrikaans and/or African languages. To ensure the reliability of the information, participants were requested to express themselves in the language with which they felt most comfortable. Translation was assured by a competent person drawn from the community. Each of the eight FGDs had between eight and ten respondents to ensure maximum interaction and participation. A total of 74 participants were involved in the FGDs in the four provinces. Three groups comprised men and women or mixed gender, while five were all-female. The discussion was loosely structured to raise answers to the following themes:

- The impact of AIDS on communities and personal experience of the epidemic,
- Knowledge and participation in local government elections,
- Expectations and perceptions of councillors' performance,
- Voluntary Counselling and Testing (VCT) and disclosure by the leadership, and
- Policy proposals on local government responses.

It should be mentioned that the responses from the FGDs could be influenced by the fact that respondents were mainly drawn from support groups and other community organisations. For this reason, participants might have a fair knowledge of the epidemic and its impact on their lives and communities.

Table 9: Focus-group construction			
	Total number of respondents	PLWHA	Marital status
FGD 1 Mixed-gender focus group: Saldanha Bay	10	data not available	Married 2 Single 2 Divorced 2 Undeclared 4
FGD 2 Mixed-gender focus group: Steinkopf	10	data not available	Married 6 Divorced 1 Widowed 1 Undeclared 2
FGD 3 Females: Ladysmith	6	data not available	Single 6
FGD 4 Females: Bergville	8	8	Married 2 Single 1 Widowed 1 Undeclared 4
FGD 5 Females: Welkom	10	10	Married 2 Single 4 Widowed 1 Undeclared 3
FGD 6 Females: Theunissen	10	data not available	Married 1 Single 6 Undeclared 3
FGD 7 Mixed-gender focus group: Springbok	10	3	Married 1 Single 1 Undeclared 8
FGD 8 Females: Piketberg	8	data not available	Married 1 Single 6 Widowed 1

FINDINGS

IMPACT OF HIV/AIDS ON COMMUNITIES

> *I have many relatives that have passed away due to AIDS. What amazes me is that so many people can die in the same family. I know this one family, where all the children died because of AIDS.* (Female, Ladysmith)

The study found that members of all eight focus groups had experienced HIV/AIDS at family and community levels, through the loss of relatives, friends and work colleagues. Generally, there was an informed expression of knowledge about the symptoms of HIV/AIDS from participants in the groups, which can be explained by their stated engagement in civic activity of one form or another.

Dominant views among participants indicated that there was a reluctance to test or disclose within their communities, which they attributed to a fear of exclusion from employment and other economic benefits. Others described their environment as hostile toward PLWHAs, a factor that they said contributed to denial. Fear of ostracism from society was openly expressed by the focus groups (some of which included PLWHAs). Participants from Ladysmith talked of denial being partly related to the tendency by employers to exclude from employment those who are infected.

Most participants, across the different age groups, indicated that unemployment, prostitution, drug use and child abuse were key drivers of the epidemic in their areas. Participants in Steinkopf, for example, indicated that their HIV/AIDS situation was compounded by prostitution, worsened by the presence of truck drivers. Because the area is en route to Namibia, some participants felt the cases of teenage pregnancy, drug use, and abuse of women and children were interconnected. Others reported that low unemployment rates played a part in fuelling dangerous behaviour. Mixed-gender focus groups expressed similar scenarios of communities burdened by sickness and orphans, all further complicated by stigma, which kept people from reporting freely to clinics for testing and treatment.

Illiteracy, intergenerational sex and poverty were cited across all groups as some of the main causes of high HIV-prevalence levels within the communities. Parental guidance and openness about HIV with children were mentioned as some ways of breaking the walls of silence and a means to ensuring an AIDS-free generation.

They reported that many teachers had died in their municipal area and that, in some instances, schools went without the required professional support.

COMMUNITY EXPECTATIONS AND PERCEPTIONS OF COUNCILLOR PERFORMANCE

Against this backdrop, the expectation of government responsibility for their welfare was generally very high among all groups. There were mixed feelings as to whether local government elections have any significant impact on people's lives. Some participants living with HIV/AIDS viewed elections as unfruitful and promoted the idea of a stay-away by all affected by the epidemic because of what they see as poor service delivery.

In Ladysmith, one participant felt officials did not care about PLWHAs. A Welkom participant thought elections could help to change things, but that elected representatives seemed to have too many contending priorities to concentrate on the real issues. The majority of Springbok participants did not think that their participation in elections could improve ordinary citizens' lives because politicians often broke their promises.

SERVICE DELIVERY

While in general terms, favourable achievements were attributed to central government, there was little reference to councillors as drivers of hope and change in relation to HIV/AIDS. In a rare show of appreciation of a representative, participants in Welkom highlighted the positive role played by a female councillor in addressing AIDS in their communities. She was reported to be active in providing support to bereaved families in the area and is hence seen to be concerned about the plight of local people.

Across focus groups, participants knew the difference between a ward councillor and a PR councillor. They all seemed to know who their ward councillors were and to which party they were affiliated. Their expectations of service delivery range from basic necessities of life, such as water and sanitation, to housing and the provision of a cure for AIDS. Across the groups, there were high expectations that government would provide food parcels and Anti-retrovirals (ARVs) to all who had HIV/AIDS. All the groups were of the opinion that support structures for HIV/AIDS had largely improved since 1994. Participants pointed to the wider availability of Anti-retroviral Therapy (ART), food parcels and social grants. However, they attributed most of the positive outcomes to non-governmental organisations (NGOs) and central government, rather than local government.

> What upsets me is that, when your CD4 count is above 200, you cannot get a government grant. I do not understand how you are going to be able to survive when you are sick, because government does no longer give people food parcels. (Female, Ladysmith)

> I think they [government] should create jobs for positive people and keep themselves busy and not just focus on ARVs … (Female, Theunissen)

> What the government is doing is not right. It is really sad when a person is sick and they do not get a grant. Their kids will go hungry. (Mixed-gender focus group, 25–70 years, Welkom)

There was some discomfort expressed about the manner in which VCT was made available to the public, particularly the mobile stations that visit localities. Some participants felt there was a lack of privacy, which served to alienate a lot of people. It was reported that community members were often afraid of being associated with HIV/AIDS should they be seen entering the mobile vans. Some of the participants did not know about VCT.

Participants in Saldanha Bay reported that the impact of AIDS had been exacerbated by ignorance, the labelling of HIV-positive people and denial. Projecting what constitutes a minority view in the focus groups, they absolved government of blame for the extent of the epidemic in their area.

> I think the government is doing a lot and I believe they are really trying to reach out to these people. I believe that, as a community, we also need to start standing up and taking responsibility for ourselves.
> (Mixed-gender focus group, Springbok)

There were further minority concerns about the likelihood that government may be overwhelmed by the wave of demand for ARVs and food parcels, and simply give up.

> I think as a black nation, we all want to take care of ourselves. Everybody looks out for their own interests. (Female, Welkom)

> … They also promise us various work-related projects, but nothing was delivered and the following (next) time you see them, they are driving posh cars …
> (Female, Piketberg)

> Well the councillor promised us that he would build houses for the people who are HIV-positive, but those were all empty promises. (Female, Welkom)

Generally, councillors were portrayed by the participants as being self-centred rather than society-centred in their execution of public affairs. The following were some of the key areas that participants expected their councillors to deliver on:

- Reducing unemployment,
- Reducing alcohol abuse (as a means of reducing dangerous behaviour),
- Involvement in awareness campaigns,
- Establishing infrastructure for trauma counselling,
- More regular interaction with communities to establish issues first-hand,
- Household surveys to clearly define the challenges communities are facing,
- Easier access to ARVs (proximity of clinics, transport),
- Establishing a specialised unit for tuberculosis patients to avoid recontamination (Springbok),
- To ensure that the social grant remains permanent and applicable to all HIV-positive people and is not limited to those with a CD4 count lower than 200, and
- To promote further research on HIV/AIDS vaccines.

> … We are asked to vote for a party and they get elected. But at the end of the day, I do not really see a big change in our community … (Female, Piketberg)

> They just come at the time of the election and then you never see them again.
> (Mixed-gender focus group, 25–70 years, Steinkopf)

> He (the ward councillor) has organised workshops that I have attended. They are very involved in workshops and they provide help with funerals. I feel that, particularly with HIV/AIDS, they are really getting involved and helping the people out. (Mixed-gender focus group, Springbok)

While there was a predominance of responses that reflected deep distrust of their councillors' ability to fulfil electioneering promises, one participant from Saldanha Bay's mixed-gender focus group suggested that the communities were too inclined to being 'spoon-fed' by the government. Another said that it is necessary to vote and accept that change does not come instantly. Some participants, underlining a minority view, stated: 'Our people don't want to stand up and do things for themselves.'

OPENNESS OF LEADERSHIP ABOUT HIV STATUS

There was consensus around the need for councillors to test and disclose their status as a way of reducing stigma and discrimination in local communities. Minority views disagreed with this position, stressing the importance of respecting confidentiality. Some participants recommended that elected officials should be allowed the freedom to maintain their silence on their personal status without undue pressure.

> I respect Mangosuthu Buthelezi for disclosing his son's status. I thought initially it is poor people like me who suffer from the disease. (Female, Ladysmith)

> I think it is important for people who are in parliament to disclose their status, because it encourages those of us who are rich if we know that even important people get this disease. (Female, Welkom)

> People have lost faith in politics, but if it was made public that one of our leaders had HIV/AIDS, it would help a lot of people, as they would think if a leader can come forward with their status, why can't they? (Female, Piketberg)

Minority opinions said, however, that communities might be reluctant to elect a candidate who has HIV owing to the notion that he or she might soon succumb to mortality and leave their needs unattended. One participant from Bergville argued that politicians should not disclose because it may project South Africa as being a doomed society: 'They should not tell because the whole country would die.'

Although some participants argued that 'people have lost faith in politics', they still believed that voting for an HIV-positive candidate would build faith in leaders in terms of their commitment to reversing the epidemic. The dominant view asserted that a community would vote for an HIV-positive person standing for councillorship, provided he or she had the right credentials.

A much more detailed study employing public opinion surveys might be useful in unravelling the extent to which HIV-positive candidates will be acceptable to the wider public. According to prior Idasa experience, the disadvantage of focus groups is that participants are likely to be swayed by dominant voices, particularly the much older members of the group. In a sense, there is the possibility that some participants may have been communicating opinions that sit well with the group dynamic. Conversely, a public opinion survey is anonymous and there is no direct contact with the interviewer, thereby providing an environment where brutally honest responses will be delivered.

While a minority expressed concern that the community would not be receptive to a candidate with HIV/AIDS, the dominant view suggested that there should be measures in government and party systems to support the emergence of leaders who have the virus. The consensus appeared to be that leaders were just as affected by HIV/AIDS as their communities. In short, there should be no pretence that HIV/AIDS afflicts only the poor.

The general impression is that we must build on the positives and ensure that more leaders 'come out' – a process that might serve to normalise HIV/AIDS, some suggest, or energise the entire campaign. There were some fears expressed that voting for a candidate with HIV would mean the community would be living with the preferred candidate for only a short time. Some saw this as problematic, particularly if the catalogue of demands needed to be met within the time spans expected by the populace.

VOTING FOR AN HIV-POSITIVE COUNCILLOR

We would vote for them. Maybe they might come up with many programmes, because he knows what is happening with positive people ... (Female, Theunissen)

I will vote for him, because people with AIDS have the same rights and we may not discriminate. (Mixed gender focus group, Steinkopf)

They (the community) will not show respect towards them. (Mixed-gender focus group, Springbok)

...If he is a good person, then I think they would support him... (Mixed-gender focus group, Saldanha Bay)

In all groups, there were participants who professed having knowledge of a councillor who might have died of HIV/AIDS, albeit without verification of the actual cause of death. We deduce from this line of reasoning that there is a strong perception among this group that people in high political office are just as affected by HIV/AIDS as the rest of the community.

CONCLUSION

The findings, as indicated earlier, represent the views of a relatively small segment of the 12 municipalities. The focus group participants are already active in their communities or in the field of HIV/AIDS, and are, therefore, expected to be better informed about issues such as stigma and discrimination. Their generally positive inclination towards voting for HIV-positive councillors could be explained by this factor.

A mixed picture emerges from these discussions. On the one hand, participants emphasise the issues associated with HIV/AIDS within their communities as constituting social ills that, ordinarily, their local authorities should be dealing with – among them, drug abuse, child abuse, unemployment and prostitution. They also suggest that, despite their communities being highly affected by HIV/AIDS, denial and a fear of disclosure permeate their societies, ostensibly due to the experience of discrimination from employment, ostracism from the community and general hostility toward PLWHAs. These opinions point to the potential for HIV/AIDS councillors to be marginalised or shunned by communities at the lower end of the literacy ladder should they disclose their status. We surmise that these barriers might cause a well-meaning representative to withdraw from quarterly meetings with local communities and lead to less accountability or less effectiveness in their functions.

On the other hand, some participants hold that elected representatives should show leadership by publicly declaring their status.

However, opinions expressed by some councillors suggest that disclosure could be potentially career threatening, indicating the complexity of this issue. The effect on careers could emanate not from society at large, but from the political party establishment that might be reluctant to sponsor an openly HIV-positive person into government. Although no clear impressions emerged from the councillors as to how political parties would respond to their status, rolling back the institutional barriers to PLWHAs' participation in decision-making might be one way of encouraging openness on HIV among the leadership.

The general impression projected by the participants is that their dire situations are expected to be reversed in great measure by their local councillors. Participants anticipate a radical change in their present circumstances, with demands for better housing, employment opportunities, social welfare and education characterising all the discussions.

Interwoven with these demands are their health needs. Most of them seemed to understand the connection between being in gainful employment and the capacity to survive HIV/AIDS, and all demands were placed in this context.

The argument for fragility, without extensive corroborating evidence, is evidently weak. If we approach it from the perspective of governance, we might be able to still suggest the position that absenteeism, due to a fear of rejection by the community, will be the most likely cause of a perceived disconnect of the relationship between a community and its councillors.

CHAPTER SIX

HOW DO MUNICIPALITIES DEAL WITH HIV/AIDS AMONG STAFF AND COUNCILLORS?

W e have witnessed trends in deaths among councillors, particularly males below the age of 50. This is indicative of what might be described as an 'abnormal' mortality profile. While there is no prima facie case established as to the cause of these deaths, the occurrence of early deaths among relatively young councillors (30–49 years) provides a basis for local authorities to critically examine the causes and craft some potential strategies if needs be.

It seems also from the interviews with councillors, that stigma does play a role in causing non-disclosure among elected representatives. This raises the possibility that some councillors may be in denial and only seek medication when it is too late for an intervention to be initiated successfully. These interventions, we would imagine, will be essential in ensuring that institutional memory is not lost over time.

The inclusion of general staff in the scope of this inquiry is based on our understanding of how local government in South Africa works. The political system relies on the administrative system to deliver on a range of set priorities. When elected representatives die, it is the administrative system that is assigned to second a ward liaison officer (working with a Proportional Representation [PR] councillor in some instances) to deal with the needs of the community in the interim period.

The chapter, therefore, in examining the mechanisms available to deal with HIV/AIDS among the rank and file of municipal councillors, extends its inquiry in some measure to professional and general staff. In making this inquiry, we attempt to understand how a response to HIV/AIDS may sustain a political system faced with the ravages of an epidemic, or how the lack of informed interventions may contribute to fragility.

THE RESPONSE FRAMEWORK

As indicated earlier, the Department of Provincial and Local Government (DPLG) released policy guidelines that provide the road map for how HIV/AIDS should be mainstreamed into all areas of local government business. The logic behind these guidelines resides in an understanding of HIV/AIDS as a social issue whose prevalence affects development (DPLG: 2007).

The DPLG framework is hinged on the concept of mainstreaming – a managerial approach to the governance of the HIV/AIDS epidemic that seeks to harness the capacities of all departments in local government to assume mutually reinforcing roles.

The DPLG document understands mainstreaming as a way of reducing everyday municipal business costs, and minimising local government's budget and capacity constraints. However, it does not seem to consider the cost implications of initial planning and training. In many municipalities it would involve shifting away from old planning and organisational models, while in others it would require the creation of new structures altogether.

In terms of the DPLG guidelines, mainstreaming HIV/AIDS takes two forms: internal and external. Both have cost implications. HIV planning is internally mainstreamed through the planning mechanisms of the Integrated Development Plan (IDP), the planning of services and the provision of Employee Assistance Programmes (EAPs). Human resource policies that provide Voluntary Counselling and Testing (VCT) and Anti-retroviral Therapy (ART) all form part of the administrative responses and internal institutional coping mechanisms dealing with HIV/AIDS.

External mainstreaming assumes that HIV will be factored into the core business of the municipality – that services will be recreated into a standard that will inhibit the exposure of HIV-positive individuals to conditions that would compromise their health and quality of life (DPLG: 2007). A related blueprint by the South African Local Government Association (SALGA) goes further and defines the roles and responsibilities of mayors, councillors, municipal managers, line function heads, IDP managers and IDP representative forums related to HIV/AIDS.

Table 10: Role player responsibilities	
Role players	Roles and responsibilities
Executive mayoral system	• leads the HIV/AIDS agenda throughout the municipality • ensures that the positions to drive the agenda are filled and function effectively
Council speaker	• ensures that ward councillors champion HIV/AIDS in their wards
Portfolio councillor	• champions HIV/AIDS in their portfolios
Ward councillor	• champions HIV/AIDS in wards with support of ward committees
Municipal manager	• ensures municipal plans, programmes and projects mainstream HIV/AIDS • ensures that programming activities cover both the workplace and community dimensions of HIV/AIDS
Line function head	• ensures municipal plans, programmes and projects mainstream HIV/AIDS in their area of functions
IDP manager	• ensures that the IDP process includes the voice of HIV/AIDS • mainstreaming is included in the IDP and monitors progress
IDP representative forum	• ensures that interest groups, communities and stakeholders they represent are able to consider and express their respective concerns on HIV/AIDS
Source: SALGA (2008).	

The framework is idealistic and, therefore, presents a properly functioning institution with knowledgeable officers who are empowered to check on one another as they ensure effective delivery of services to People Living With HIV and AIDS (PLWHAs).

FINDINGS

The summary of findings related to the institutional responses of 12 municipal areas in four provinces are as follows:

PRESENCE OF POLICIES

With the exception of two, all municipalities indicated they had a policy to deal with HIV/AIDS. In Bergrivier (Piketberg), no policy was mentioned, and in Ladysmith/Bergville (Emnambithi-Ladysmith/Okhahlamba), the municipalities had outsourced the drafting of their policies to an external service provider.

ART

It was reported that ART was available through clinics and medical aid structures. Municipalities admitted no direct control over the provision of ARV medication.

ABSENTEEISM

With the exception of Piketberg, all the municipalities admitted that absenteeism was a growing issue among workers in the lower salary grades. It was also cited as a growing concern among senior professional staff in the administrative system in Theunissen. Councillors tended to avoid using council medical services, presumably due to fear of the public discovering their HIV status.

ORGANISATIONAL IMPACT

HIV was widely believed to have an economic impact on municipalities in terms of rental income and the collection of rates and taxes. HIV/AIDS programmes, such as local AIDS councils, were mentioned in Ladysmith and Theunissen as being costly to implement because capacity-building and training had to be done to get councillors and staff up to speed with HIV-prevention and -awareness campaigns. In the smaller municipalities of the Western Cape, it was generally thought that HIV would have no impact on organisational ability. These were the exceptions; the balance noted some form of HIV-related impact or the start thereof.

The application of policy and the availability of resources to deal with HIV/AIDS appear uneven across municipalities. Bearing this in mind, and to insulate themselves from the effects of staff shortages and declining productivity, municipalities have existing structures to aid them. Medical aids, as a cost to municipality, ART and absenteeism, all combine to stress tax resources.

MEDICAL AIDS

According to the interviewees, medical aid schemes are available in the public sector, although somewhat unevenly across grade scales. Councillors may belong to medical aids on a voluntary basis, but the contributions are taken directly from their allowances.

Many medical aids make provision for ART, although it is not clear which ones do and which ones do not as medical aid conditions differ from package to package, across schemes and across municipal boundaries. The IDP manager for Springbok informed us that medical aids are voluntary, whereas other municipalities suggested medical aid was compulsory for all employees, with the municipality paying 60% of the total contribution. The salary grades to which medical aids are applicable were not specified, although the state does make provision for free basic health care and ART for those who meet the criteria.

Councillors in the wards were allowed to voluntarily take medical insurance and select their own benefits, depending on their personal needs. The availability of medical aids, therefore, does not ensure that all councillors are covered for ART. However, many municipalities did have clinics where ART could be sourced. In Warrenton it was disclosed that, '… two [councillors] are using their medical aids because they are not free to be seen in public collecting [ART] medication'.

Again, even within institutions, people are influenced by wider society and its attitude towards HIV/AIDS. This also influences the cost to the municipality. If ART is procured through a clinic, the cost is borne by the province; if it is accessed through a medical aid, the cost is partly borne by the municipality. Some officials made sweeping generalisations that cannot explain the reluctance of ART uptake among senior and junior staff.

If 'everybody has access to anti-retroviral treatment', the HIV coordinator in Welkom suggested, we are still left with the issue of stigma and the constancy of ART supplies at clinics. Norms governing disclosure and treatment very much influence the uptake of ART and how it occurs. There is no conclusive data to support this claim; at this stage it is merely anecdotal evidence.

The municipal manager in Richards Bay mentioned that, at the lower salary scale of the staff compliment, '[W]e do not keep information as to how many people we have employed, because we have lost plenty of people due to AIDS … [W]e identify people, we counsel people and we keep matters of people private … If people have AIDS, it remains a secret. We provide medicines and support services.'

This can be problematic as we have already seen anecdotal evidence that some people perceive testing is not an option because of a larger denialism in society. If testing is not an option, Anti-retrovirals (ARVs) are not being applied to their greatest potential. The HIV/AIDS coordinator in Welkom alludes to this: 'Those that agree to test are being tested, and each and every client [receives] a certificate of test. From there you will be referred respectively and those that qualify for ARVs will be referred to ARV sites … but with the stigma that is hanging around in people's minds, we are unable to achieve that.'

In Warrenton, the HIV officer supports this claim, saying that, '[M]any people are dying without knowing their status. Since I started in 2005, I would say that three people died of AIDS.'

While the unwillingness to disclose forms part of the issue, it has also been acknowledged that ART and the issues surrounding stigma contribute to the lack of ART uptake. Even where there is a willingness to disclose and go onto the ART regimen, logistical issues are raised in some of the more remote areas. In Bergville, the municipal manager observed that, '… people know that there is a disease called HIV out there. The only problem now is how do we distribute or get the ARV throughout our rural communities?'

ABSENTEEISM: A POSSIBLE INDICATOR OF PREVALENCE

One of the influences identified with the policy of non-disclosure and voluntary testing is information deficit. An HIV coordinator raised this issue. If people remain silent on something as severe as HIV/AIDS, then one cannot benchmark one's progress in dealing with it institutionally or socially. At this juncture, the organisational influence of HIV/AIDS on capacity is difficult to measure in the absence of reliable attendance records.

The IDP managers in Springbok and Ladysmith, and the municipal manager of Richards Bay, all identify people in the lower salary grades as susceptible to HIV/AIDS.

If one sees it thus, the generalisation that HIV is a disease of the semi-skilled and poor appears to be reinforced, but the stigma and silence around HIV make this assertion difficult to prove.

> [HIV/AIDS] … has really affected a lot of people … we have been faced with a lot of absenteeism. Office productivity won't be here and then we need to deal with stigma … you would rather stay home because you won't want to see those people tomorrow. (HIV coordinator, Welkom)

> I think we have not reached a stage where we say that people are falling per day, but we are reaching a phase where people are becoming more frequently ill than what they used to prior to the epidemic. And if there is a programme in place, and whoever has been facilitating the programme is not healthy, of course that programme will not continue. (IDP manager, Theunissen)

Indirectly, absenteeism and sustained capacity issues can indicate the presence of HIV in the workforce. We could possibly also include early retirements and sudden resignations following prolonged and frequent absenteeism as indicators of HIV's impact on institutional capacity and councillors alike.

The results of capacity being influenced by HIV-induced absenteeism are mixed. Municipalities indicate that planning is affected in ways beyond their control – two noted aspects being population fluctuations and absenteeism. Transient populations affect municipalities differently and may affect costs seasonally, just as monitoring population movements may aid in better HIV planning.

Internally, however, capacity is affected because the ill will not put in their expected share of work or report regularly for duty.

> [Y]ou get a number of absentee people who cannot come to work because they are sick, suffering from pneumonia, suffering from TB, suffering from meningitis, stiffness in the neck; we have got a number, in fact we have got a system where we've got workers who are not part of our employment, but who are called relief workers who are on standby, so that we call them and say come and assist when we reach this position where we feel we don't have enough workforce … [to ensure] our positions are fully filled … because of the epidemic we have these relief workers to assist in order to address the challenge. (IDP manager, Theunissen)

In the Theunissen municipality, the fluctuation in illness and its severity has caused the local authority to increase its labour costs because it has to recruit a 'reserve labour force' to step into the breach when illness and HIV-related medical conditions cause absenteeism.

However, the municipal managers in Richards Bay and Piketberg both thought their capacity had not yet been affected. The tone of the phrasing is apt:

We have always been lucky; we are never affected in terms of sustainability. We have a well-run and capacitated municipality.
(Municipal manager, Richards Bay)

Absenteeism is being addressed by responsive deployment. In Springbok, workers were being multi-skilled to minimise the costs and effects of absenteeism. In two municipalities, it was noted that workers infected with HIV were being given lighter work to keep them employed and to minimise the community effect of a worker and his family becoming instantly pauperised by HIV/AIDS. Unfortunately, light work assignments also have the effect of slowing down services and may deepen the community sense of 'nothing being done'.

The textured nature of prevalence denies concrete patterns that cut across municipalities and are difficult to measure. An IDP manager makes this point well when he says, '... one cannot stand up scientifically and say yes [HIV affects the municipality] in this way. I have noticed a considerable number of absentees from [within the ranks of] key role players in the municipality, because they are sick.'

Some municipalities feel the effects of HIV more readily than others due to a number of reasons beyond the scope of this study. Transient labour, seasonal employment opportunities and the depth of social stigmatisation associated with HIV/AIDS all seem to compound existing issues in service delivery and in providing ART to contain the institutional effects of these drivers of HIV/AIDS.

Even if the human element was to take care of itself, and there was no noticeable HIV/AIDS impact on productivity and sustainability, containing the issue in broader society would present significant challenges. For example, many municipalities cite issues with budgeting as being of grave concern.

Within the local governance mandate to promote employment and development, the chair of the Saldanha Bay council's finance committee noted that their 2006/7 capital expenditure budget had declined from R25 million (US$3,3 million) to R10 million (US$1,3 million) – a fact reinforced in the IDP reports for the same period. Many of the councils in this study may not have felt the same decline in revenue.

Respondents indicated that HIV and its related effects are likely to accelerate economic stress in councils. Municipalities in this study have noted that they take responsibility for awareness and training, as per their mandate. The IDP manager in Theunissen noted that the epidemic has created a heightened need and urgency to plough resources into HIV awareness, training and education.

In Ladysmith, the IDP manager made it clear, through his observations on ward capacity, that SALGA mandates could not be fully implemented, nor attention be given to DPLG mainstreaming initiatives, due to resource constraints.

The DPLG mainstreaming framework implies SALGA knowledge systems were already in place and that local government merely had to incorporate new policy into existing practise.

Those structures, local AIDS councils, the ward AIDS councils ... we have to bring those structures together and that has cost us a lot. We had a workshop for those structures; we have spent around R30 000. (IDP manager, Ladysmith)

Income streams in municipalities, as a result of HIV, declined due to the severity of the epidemic within those communities. The IDP managers in Theunissen and Ladybrand acknowledged this.

> *Now that we've got this epidemic of HIV/AIDS, of course, each municipality would be running excessive training and community awareness, so you've got more money going into training, whether it is about being infected or affected, in terms of HIV education.* (IDP manager, Theunissen)

The cost to council increases with the spread of the epidemic, some respondents said. Not only is more spent on training and education, but the revenue base declines to cope with the epidemic. This means that grant income allocations, which all municipalities in this study receive would have to increase to offset shortfalls between municipal revenue and expenditure.

Two examples of income stream loss are worth noting. The IDP manager in Ladybrand observes that, '… [I]n areas where we have people who are infected by HIV/AIDS, the majority of them are not working and are poor, and we have had to provide free basic services like electricity, water and sanitation, irrespective of whether that person is working or not. That places a financial burden on the council … We have got a hospital full of people with HIV/AIDS and, as a council, we had to sacrifice that building which is a very valuable building. It was an area we would normally rent out.'

In some instances, and in terms of rates and taxes and rental income, HIV might contribute gradually to the impoverishment of local government structures. This could weaken the ability of councillors to become agents of development, because their main partners in service delivery – the administrative and financial systems of local government – would gradually run out of resources.

CONCLUSION

While much of the information in this chapter relates to the administrative system of local government, it gives an impression, in qualitative terms, of how poor performance at this level might undermine the political role of councillors who rely on this segment of local government to implement policy.

The general impression is that municipalities have to adapt to a changing human context by devising ways of being effective amidst absenteeism caused by illnesses.

Municipal areas are evidently compromised by the lack of a holistic HIV policy to guide their responses. Internally, respondents noted the presence of EAP and VCT initiatives. Overall, progress was regarded as inadequate as many staff fall prisoner to the same fears held by people in the wider community.

We find that councillors are provided access to medical schemes or encouraged to voluntarily enlist for alternative schemes. While VCT and ART are generally available, there is a perceived reluctance by councillors to test and know their HIV status, due to a fear of being judged in the public eye – a stigma-induced response, it would seem. This behaviour limits the capacity of council planners to determine the extent of ART uptake and is an impediment to effective responses to the epidemic.

From the interviews, it was unclear as to the stage of development local AIDS councils had progressed. In some areas it was clear from the focus groups that no progress had been made, as communities had had no contact with any councillors bearing such news. Capacity was an issue and knowledge availability another. One senior manager from Ladybrand made it clear that council resources were being invested in training people in the local and ward AIDS councils.

In half of the municipalities, the presence and activities of ward AIDS councils and local AIDS councils were noted, but this study did not determine their degree of functionality. It was also noted that responsibility and accountability for awareness was not clearly demarcated. HIV/AIDS awareness and education programmes were determined as being run from the clinic – a district or provincial responsibility. However, some councillors and managers do not acknowledge AIDS awareness as a local responsibility. The general trend is that AIDS initiatives are viewed as political and, therefore, given to the mayor's office to be run from a special programmes portfolio.

This implies that mainstreaming is not occurring, and many managers and councillors believe that HIV/AIDS should have a greater budget share, even though its extent has not been quantified. Direct budgeting was, therefore, regarded as a more effective means of confronting HIV – a sensibility that runs against the DPLG mainstreaming proposals.

RECOMMENDATIONS

IDENTIFYING CHAMPIONS

A deliberate effort needs to be made to identify champions among the councillors in local government who could form the core of leadership dedicated to mainstreaming HIV/AIDS into the administrative and political systems of local authorities. Such an intervention would require involving the political party establishments represented in local government to embrace a common approach for all their councillors, to ensure longevity, consistency and continuity.

CAPACITY FOR THE RIGHT PEOPLE

Capacity building on mainstreaming and community organising skills should primarily target technical staff (HIV/AIDS managers, municipal managers, IDP managers). HIV training for councillors, driven by empowered and relevant technical staff, would ensure that councillors are equipped to handle the needs of communities afflicted with HIV/AIDS. This would also ensure a more sustained institutional capacity to deal with HIV.

LEADERSHIP

Leadership visibility and consistent communication and advocacy on prevention, treatment, care and support among representatives, is likely to keep HIV/AIDS on the political agenda for the foreseeable future. However, such programmes require the strategic support of specialist NGOs and developmental agencies, which could serve as partners of poorly capacitated municipal councils.

ALLEVIATE THE STRESS OF HIV TESTING

Wellness programmes to look after the general health of employees and councillors would not only assist in determining who is ill with the more severe ailments, but also identify people who require specialised treatment. They would maintain the confidentiality of usual medical interactions supplied by VCT, without the pressure or fear of knowingly going for such a test. Regular medical check-ups for councillors are therefore recommended, rather than VCT alone, which has its limitations. This might reduce the number of councillors dying in denial.

CREATE BROADER INSTITUTIONAL OWNERSHIP OF HIV

HIV is not a core function in the Project Consolidate framework. HIV is also largely regarded as a political question solved through mayoral offices and council health committees, which do not always transmit capacity to the ward councillors to deal with the needs of their constituents. Treating HIV/AIDS as a special project of political concern would account for the lack of capacity to mainstream HIV into core municipal business as conceptualised by the DPLG mainstreaming framework.

DISCLOSURE AND 'POLITICAL STIGMA'

Running public opinion surveys that answer the question 'Would you vote for someone who has HIV?' would help to boost social morale and contribute to 'normalising' HIV/AIDS in the eyes of the community. If the opinion surveys confirm that people are prepared to vote for HIV-positive people who prove effective in their mandates, it may encourage more elected leaders to disclose. Disclosure would facilitate ART uptake by reducing stigma. This would increase the working life of technical staff and councillors, and lessen the impression that voting for an HIV-positive person is not worth it.

Research

Municipalities generally lack databases and research capacity. Established research units will be useful for effective planning. Information on staff attrition to AIDS hence remains largely anecdotal and may compromise effective planning. To measure effective government, accountability and legitimacy, researchers will need to have access to attendance registers, minutes of council meetings and records that relate to service delivery. From the experience of this project and related projects undertaken by Idasa, many of these records are either poorly stored or not easily accessible.

CHAPTER SEVEN

REFLECTING ON OUTCOMES AND UNANSWERED QUESTIONS

Despite its stated limitations, this project unravels some key pointers to a nation haemorrhaged by unnatural deaths among relatively young citizens, the trends of which mimic the AIDS mortality profile. Different scenarios are presented that might inform the notion of fragility as occasioned by HIV/AIDS. The first is that the high rates of deaths among councillors is likely to compromise South Africa's ability to build an experienced corps of politicians at local level. Members of Parliament will sometimes be drawn from this pool of people, who would incrementally improve their record of performance at grassroots level. Similar impacts on the administrative system, combined with other pre-existing causes of skills attrition, as suggested anecdotally in the research, might contribute to ineffective government.

The shortage of skilled personnel and their constant loss to other sectors; the anecdotal evidence reported by respondents regarding absenteeism; illnesses and deaths among the general workforce, councillors and professionals are all indicative of a silent but worrying impression of institutional incapacity in South Africa's local government structures.

The failures to harness skills and deliver services are already well documented by the government's own Project Consolidate. We view this as an admission by central government of weak governance at local level.

By all indications, these weaknesses persisted beyond 2006. Despite this, the Department of Provincial and Local Government (DPLG) framework on AIDS and local governance expects municipalities to play a pivotal role in the fight against the epidemic. This appears unrealistic in our view, given all the capacity issues that may or may not be wrought by HIV/AIDS. The question of institutional weakness is one to be further explored.

Certainly the combined effect of resignations and deaths among councillors is having an impact on the complexion of local government in terms of ruling party-opposition power relations. While it seems the opposition has generally tended to lose most by-elections, the ruling ANC has had positive growth recording a net gain of 31 seats from by-elections held between 2001 and 2006. There is nothing undemocratic about this scenario.

However, it needs to be stated that it is highly unlikely for political parties outside of parliament to compete effectively in these polls, because of the financial and organisational challenges associated with by-elections. We recall that the criteria for allocating state financing is based on the proportion of parliamentary seats held by a given political party. Even among the parties with access to these resources, it is the larger parties that reap the most benefit, albeit well-earned through open competition.

While the weaknesses of the opposition in South Africa is well noted at national level, local government is a terrain that tends to be more competitive, particularly in the Western Cape and KwaZulu-Natal. This tier of government hence presents smaller parties with a realistic opportunity to dominate decision-making processes. The loss of elected representatives by small parties will continue to cause them to lose policy influence in local government for as long as they fail to retain the gains of previous elections.

From a response perspective, while in principle AIDS should be a key performance area, in practice it does not appear to be considered a core mandate of the municipalities. Municipalities in this study present a picture of desperation in terms of how they handle this. Their knowledge of mainstreaming is weak, and policies are in place in some, but not all, local authorities.

The political leaders, the ward councillors, interviewed in this study, profess to need training and new knowledge on how to deal effectively with the myriad issues faced by their constituencies. And yet, in the same vein, they express fears about Voluntary Counselling and Testing (VCT) and disclosure. How, then, could they be expected to take a leading role?

The levels of denial, we argue, may contribute to the unusually high number of deaths among young councillors. We get a sense that stigma and discrimination drive the AIDS-sick underground and, when they do surface, they are likely to be beyond help. While medical aid and other facilities are available within municipalities, fear of exposure to the public eye seems to limit the uptake of Anti-retrovirals (ARVs) by leaders and staff alike.

If no stopgap measures are applied to deal with community issues, absenteeism and vacancies may contribute to perceptions of non-delivery. Indirectly, this builds on an existing negative perception of local government among expectant publics.

Against a recent background of violent protests, reportedly triggered by poor service delivery, local government cannot afford not to perform. Afrobarometer studies tell us that confidence levels in local government are declining, particularly among the historically disadvantaged. They tell us that councillors are blamed for poor services when things go wrong.

DEFINING FRAGILITY MEASUREMENTS

The study obviously falls short of measuring the impact of HIV/AIDS on municipalities as this was not its stated ambition. It does, however, provide in our view a fairly compelling evidence-based argument about why AIDS will be the main explanation for attrition among elected representatives and their constituencies. It frames mortality within a context of fragility and, in some respects, governance, by discussing how these findings might affect effectiveness, accountability and legitimacy.

Future undertakings will do well to embark on the more time-consuming approaches that seek to measure the impact of AIDS on governance and, therefore, provide a more holistic illustration of the same. Such measurement would rely, in part, on:

- tracking attendance records of deceased councillors in council sessions for a specified period
- tracking reasons for and frequency of absenteeism by councillors and support staff
- obtaining and analysing records of qualifications of councillors, work experience and tangible policy contributions to local communities
- content analysis of the Hansard or equivalent to determine the nature of contributions by deceased councillors to debates
- records on uptake of ARV by councillors.

Our experience of this project suggests that this will be a challenging task given the paucity of records, the supposed propensity to avoid VCT and ART by councillors, and potential cultural and ethical considerations that might impede researchers from correlating deaths to AIDS and governance benchmarks.

HYPOTHESES

The key hypotheses requiring testing are framed in three different ways. Though related, each has an additional dimension that will compliment the others. They all respond to the vexing notion of 'political stigma', which is an ill-defined term that we have related to the reluctance of elected officials to test and disclose their HIV status. Our sense is that we should go a little further in this inquiry to understand how withdrawal affects public confidence in leadership, and in VCT and ART more generally. We have discussed in fair detail how this phenomenon could be associated with a lack of effectiveness or account-ability in governance.

HYPOTHESIS 1: THE DISCOURSE ON AIDS AND POVERTY HAS CONTRIBUTED TO DENIAL AMONG THE POLITICAL ELITE

Effects on career and the loss of livelihood are among the most serious personal issues councillors have tended to consider in their answers on personal disclosure. Such denial-ism may lead to the stigmatisation of others thought to be the most likely carriers of HIV. Further, this can lead to political (self) exclusion of councillors who may exhibit charac-teristics of the disease, such as rapid weight loss, frequent coughing and loss of vitality, all of which could be attributable to insomnia, TB, polluted environments, communicable diseases, non life-threatening sexually transmitted infections, or inadequate nutrition.

Despite the high mortality in the most affected age brackets, there has been a low re-corded uptake of ART among councillors at state-run clinics. Evidence for this was found in one municipality (Warrenton), where councillors with HIV avoided the clinic's Anti-retroviral Therapy (ART) programme and made use of their medical aids to avoid public scrutiny. A lack of willingness among political leaders to declare their status may under-mine their ability to publicly address HIV as a collectively and personally serious issue. An underlying refrain seems to suggest that HIV/AIDS is a disease of the poor and should not be associated with persons in higher income brackets, which includes politicians.

HYPOTHESIS 2: THE DENIAL AMONG POLITICAL ELITES HAS CONTRIBUTED TO NEGATIVE PUBLIC PERCEPTIONS OF ELECTED LEADERS AS CHAMPIONS OF HIV

Many participants in the focus groups expected politicians to provide leadership on HIV/AIDS, but were by and large sceptical about their commitment. The post-mortem dis-closures of political leaders on the mortality of relatives were noticed, but it was also remarked that national leaders disclose only when the HIV test results are negative. HIV-positive public disclosures were never made, except in one instance. This has led some of the councillors to declare that, should political leaders disclose their positive status, it would be a morale booster for those who consider themselves poor and marginalised. It may lend more awareness about the 'normality' of HIV, or perhaps contribute to more positive public attitudes toward VCT and ART uptake in communities, where stigma is widespread.

Councillors in this study were open about a public discussion on HIV. While willing to engage in the public discussion, personally they are not generally willing to disclose personal health details for a number of reasons: opposition politicians using the information in elections and a loss of electoral support. These fears may undermine the moral force of their contribution to minimising the impact HIV/AIDS may make on local government and communities.

HYPOTHESIS 3: A POLITICAL PUBLIC-SERVICE CAMPAIGN BASED ON THE PUBLIC TESTING AND DISCLOSURE OF ELECTED OFFICIALS MAY ASSIST IN REDUCING DISCRIMINATION TOWARDS THOSE INFECTED WITH HIV

A denialist attitude is not limited to the political elite, but can also be found in the broader population. According to an ongoing Human Sciences Research Council (HSRC) HIV-testing and behavioural survey, antenatal clinics are the major source of HIV/AIDS prevalence data. Access to private health care makes it difficult to determine prevalence among affluent sectors of the population and those with access to private health care. This has led to a false sense of security among population groups with low officially reported prevalence statistics. A common response among prospective respondents in the HSRC survey was to 'go down the road to the squatter settlement' (see, for example, Claire Keaton's 'Wealthy Restrict AIDS Researchers', *Sunday Times* 21/09/2008, and Verashni Pillay's 'News24 HIV Study: Whites, Indians Wary').

Locally elected officials express fears of social and political exclusion. A minority expressed concern about being beaten at the polls as the electorate may think that one HIV-positive person equates to an infected party that will not be able to deliver on services.

CONCLUSION

The relationship between AIDS, leadership and governance is obviously a complex one, and will continue to be a work-in-progress for researchers in this area. The related notion of fragility challenges researchers to unlock some of the doors that have previously been closed to outside inquiry.

In this regard, we underline that the information on mortality among elites and voters is sensitive, and will evidently need to be used carefully to generate the relevant policy interest and achieve set outcomes. Impact studies on strategic institutions are sometimes seen to be highly intrusive and of a security nature, thereby inhibiting the ability of researchers to understand the extent to which this epidemic affects the higher echelons of society.

There is, however, no doubt in our minds that the policy relevance of these studies is beginning to register among many influential policy agents in Africa and beyond as matters of leadership in HIV/AIDS come into sharper relief (see Chirambo: 2008). Certainly our experience in eight countries now indicates that a participatory approach – that is, the involvement of the political institutions that are being investigated in planning and review processes – has tended to allay fears of misuse of information and its relevance to the broader fight against HIV/AIDS.

This particular project, we think, serves to contribute to an expanded understanding of how AIDS might affect leadership effectiveness, accountability and legitimacy in local government in South Africa. We see it as potentially unlocking the debate around disclosure, VCT and ART for those in high office, and whether or not current approaches are helpful in rolling back stigma and discrimination.

We also see it as potentially contributing to the overall understanding of the capacity, or lack thereof, of local government to address the myriad challenges that are wrought largely by HIV/AIDS. The knowledge gaps among people entrusted to decide on AIDS priorities appear to be large. The actual engagement between councillors and communities is not fully researched, but on the basis of anecdotes seems somewhat limited. The means for implementation appear compromised by political, administrative and financial weaknesses. If this report is read in conjunction with others, such as the Auditor-General's report, the evidence becomes compelling.

The project suggests more in-depth studies are needed to measure the nature of fragility in local government, which will require an intensive collaborative exercise with local authorities to make the best of existing records on human resources, council deliberations and attendance, minutes of ward committee meetings and situational analyses, clinic records, financial data where it exists and updated municipal-level prevalence information. The cooperation of government institutions and the DPLG in particular would be most appropriate and beneficial for all.

ENDNOTES

1	Department of Provincial and Local Government History of Local Government: http://www.thedplg. gov.za/policy/?q=node/27. Retrieved 17 September 2008.

2	Ibid.

3	Calculated at an average exchange rate of R7.50 to US$1.00.

4	The following elements define 'resilience' in the context of Idasa-GAP:

- That all institutions have a working knowledge of the political, economic and social dynamics of HIV/AIDS, and that this is reflected in their policy/strategy documents.

- That new knowledge and strategies are integrated into education and knowledge systems to strengthen the capacity of our youth and communities to deal with the disease.

- That state and non-state actors develop a culture of common problem-solving and collaborative actions.

- That stigma and discrimination are weeded out at all levels of society (unlock the walls around stigma at all levels).

- That People Living With HIV and AIDS (PLWHAs) participate in decision-making mechanisms on HIV/AIDS and other governance priorities (participation in leadership not based on HIV status).

- That the content of policies and development plans continue to place HIV/AIDS as one of our biggest challenges.

- That our leaders are not only involved, but also seen to be involved in HIV/AIDS work at a strategic level, as well as local, community, national and regional levels (e.g. Coalition of African Parliamentarians Against HIV and AIDS [CAPAH], AIDS Councils).

- That there is universal access to quality health care and Anti-retroviral Therapy (ART) for all who need it, and that there is consensus around this (currently there is privileged health care for political leaders who, for example, may be flown out of South Africa to Europe for treatment).

5	This background is largely summarised from Idasa's *How Local Government Works: Participants' Workbook* (2006).

6	Estimates by the Department of Health and the Actuarial Society of South Africa for the period 2001–2007 show double-digit HIV-prevalence rates for the provinces named here.

7	Electoral Institute of Southern Africa: Party Political Funding: http://www.eisa.org.za/WEP/soupar- ties2b.htm. Retrieved 17 September 2008.

8	HIV/AIDS Stigma Resource Pack (n.d.).

9	The name and the location of this councillor have been withheld due to ethical concerns.

BIBLIOGRAPHY

Abdelatif, A. (2003) *Good governance and its relationship to democracy and economic development.* UNDP: South Korea. Retrieved 2008/07/24 from http://www.undp-pogar.org/publications/governance/aa/goodgov.pdf

Bond, P. (2002) *Local economic development debates in South Africa.* Retrieved 2008/05/20 from http://www.queensu.ca/msp/pages/Project_Publications/Series/6.htm#Introduction:%20A%20new%20paradigm%20for%20LED

Bratton, M. & Sibanyoni, M. (2006) 'Delivery or Responsiveness? A popular scorecard of local government performance in South Africa' Paper No. 62 Idasa: Pretoria

Callahan, K. (2007) Elements of Effective Governance: Measurement, Accountability and Participation. Rutgers University: New Jersey

Carment, D., Prest, S. & Samy, Y. (2007) 'Assessing Fragility: Theory, evidence and policy' in *Politorbis* 42(1)

Chirambo, K. (2005) HIV/AIDS and Democratic Governance in Africa, Illustrating the Impact on Electoral Processes, Idasa: Pretoria

Centre for the Study of AIDS (n.d.) *HIV/AIDS Stigma Resource Pack.* University of Pretoria: Pretoria

Chirambo, K. (2006) *Democratisation in the Age of HIV/AIDS: Understanding the political implications.* Idasa: Pretoria

Chirambo, K. (2008) *The Political Cost of AIDS: An Overview.* Idasa: Pretoria

Department for International Development (DFID) (2005) *Why We Need to Work More Effectively in Fragile States.* DFID: London

Department of Health (2008) *The National HIV and Syphilis Prevalence Survey 2007.* Department of Health

Department of Provincial and Local Government (DPLG) (2007) *Framework for an Integrated Local Response to HIV/AIDS.* DPLG: Tshwane

Dorrington, R., Bradshaw, D., Johnson, L. & Budlender, D. (2004) *The Demographic Impact of HIV/AIDS in South Africa: National and Provincial Indicators.* Department of Health, ASSA: Cape Town

Electoral Institute of Southern Africa (EISA) (2007) Funding of Political Parties. Retrieved 03/10/2008 from http://www.eisa.org.za/EISA/publications/publications.htm

Electoral Institute of Southern Africa (EISA) (2006) South Africa: Political Party Funding. Retrieved 03/10/2008 from http://www.eisa.org.za/WEP/souparties2.htm

Fourie, P. (2003) 'Global Change' in *Peace and Security* 19(3), October, pp. 281-300

Hannan, U. and Besada, H. (2007) Dimensions of State Fragility: A Review of the Social Science Literature. Working Paper 33. Retrieved 03/10/2008 from http://www.igloo.org/library/edocuments?id={29FA0A15-B4B5-455E-95AF-754C50292B7B}&view=full

Health Economics and HIV/AIDS Research Division (HEARD) (2003) *HIV Mainstreaming: A definition, some experiences and strategies.* University of Natal: Durban

Idasa (2006) *How Local Government Works: Participants' Workbook*. Local Government Centre: Pretoria

Isandla (2007) *Local Government's Responses to HIV/AIDS: A case study of the City of Cape Town's HIV/AIDS/TB multi-sectoral strategy*. Isandla: Cape Town

Jennings, R. (2002) *Discrimination and HIV/AIDS: S&T/ALP Research into the Nature and Extent of HIV Discrimination*. Department of Health: South Africa

Johannesburg Council (2004) *Chapter nine institutional arrangements*. Retrieved 2008/09/23 from http://www.joburg-archive.co.za/2004/budget/ch9.pdf

Joint Initiative on Priority Skills Acquisition Report on Activities in 2007 (2008) Office of the Deputy President of South Africa. Retrieved 3/10/2008 from http://www.info.gov.za/View/Downloadfileaction?Id=80103%20

Joseph, S. (2007) 'Building "positive" spaces: Sustainable human settlements in the context of HIV/AIDS' in *The Local Government Transformer*. October/November

Kelly, K. (2004). *South African Cities and HIV/AIDS: Challenges and Responses*. SACN: Johannesburg

Mathoho, M. (2006). *Grasping the nettle: facing the challenges of HIV/AIDS on service delivery and local governance*. CPS Policy Brief 42. Center for Policy Studies: Johannesburg

McNabb, D. (2004) Research methods for political science. M.E. Sharpe: New York

Mfecane, S. & Skinner, D. (2004) 'Stigma, discrimination and the implications for people living with HIV/AIDS' in *South Africa Journal of Social Aspects of HIV/AIDS* 1(3), November, pp. 157-164

Mnyanda, Y. (2006) *Managing HIV and AIDS Stigma in the Workplace: A case study of the Eastern Cape Department of Social Development*. Stellenbosch University: Stellenbosch

Mouton, J. & Marais, H.C. (1996) *Basic Concepts in the Methodology of the Social Sciences*. HSRC: Pretoria

Ogden, L. & Nyblade, J. (2005) *Common at its Core: HIV-related stigma across contexts*. ICRW: Washington

Parker, R. & Aggleton, P. (2003) *Social Science & Medicine* 57(1), July, pp. 13-24

Parsons, W. (1995) *Public Policy: An introduction to the theory and practice of policy analysis*. Edward Edgar Publishing Ltd: Cheltenham

IOM. (2005) Partnership on HIV and Mobility in Southern Africa (PHAMSA). Retrieved 2008/10/03 from http://iom.org.za/site/index.php?option=com_content&task=view&id=55&Itemid=60

Pillay, V. (2008) News24 HIV Study: Whites, Indians Wary. Retrieved 2008/09/22 from http://article.wn.com/view/2008/09/18/HIV_study_Whites_Indians_wary/

Politicsweb (2008) *South Africa's municipal accounts in a mess*. Retrieved 2008/08/11 from http://www.politicsweb.co.za/politicsweb/view/politicsweb/en/page72308?oid=92334&sn=Marketingweb+detail

Project Consolidate (2004) *A hands-on local government engagement programme*. Retrieved 2008/05/20 from http://www.projectconsolidate.gov.za

Rice, S. & Patrick, S. (2008) *Index of State Weakness in the Developing World*. Brookings Institute: Washington

Rousseau, J. *The social contract or principles of political right*. Retrieved 2008/08/13 from http://www.constitution.org/jjr/socon.htm

Schedler, A., Diamond, L. and Plattner, M. (1999) The Self-restraining State: Power and Accountability in New Democracies. Lynne Reiner: Colorado

Simmons, A. (2001) *Justification and Legitimacy*. Cambridge University Press: Cambridge

Shefer, T. (2004) *Gendered Representations of HIV/AIDS and the Reproduction of Hegemonic Discourses on Femininity in Media Images*. University of the Western Cape: Cape Town

South Africa Info. *Health care in South Africa*. Retrieved 2008/05/22 from http://www.southafrica.info/about/health/health.htm

South African Local Government Association (SALGA) (2008) *Country Guidelines on HIV and AIDS for Local Government*. SALGA:Tshwane

Statistics South Africa (SSA) (Census 2001) Employment Statistics. Retrieved 03/10/2008 from http://www.statssa.gov.za/timeseriesdata/pxweb2006/Dialog/varval.asp?ma=Employment%20status%20by%20District%20Council&ti=Table%3A+Census+2001+by+district+council%2C+sex%2C+employment+status++%28official+definition%29+and+population+group%2E+&path=../Database/South%20Africa/Population%20Census/Census%202001%20-%20Demarcation%20boundaries%20as%20at%2010%20October%202001/District%20Council%20level%20-%20Persons/&lang=1

Statistics South Africa (SSA) (Census 2001) Population Retrieved 03/10/2008 from http://www.statssa.gov.za/timeseriesdata/pxweb2006/Dialog/varval.asp?ma=Age%20single%20years%20by%20district%20council.&ti=Table%3A+Census+2001+by+district+council%2C+sex%2C+population+group+and++age%2E&path=../Database/South%20Africa/Population%20Census/Census%202001%20-%20Demarcation%20boundaries%20as%20at%2010%20October%202001/District%20Council%20level%20-%20Persons/&lang=1

Stebbins, R. (2001) *Exploratory Research in the Social Sciences*. Sage: California

Strand, P. & Chirambo, K. (eds) (2005) *HIV/AIDS and Democratic Governance in South Africa: Illustrating the impact on the electoral process*. Idasa: Pretoria

Swartz, L. & Roux, N. (2004) 'A study of local government HIV/AIDS projects in South Africa' in *Journal of Social Aspects of HIV/AIDS* 1(2), August

Tlakula, P. (2007) IEC presentation On Local Government Elections 2006. Retrieved 2008-08-13 from www.elections.org.za/multistakeholderconference/DocumentView.aspx?pklDocumentID=75

Tshwane Ward Committee By-laws (n.d.) Retrieved 2008-09-12 from http://www.tshwane.gov.za/documents/bylaws/bylaw_wardcommitees.pdf

UNAIDS/WHO (2006) *2006 Report on the Global AIDS Epidemic*. Retrieved 2008-03-25 from http://www.unaids.org/en/KnowledgeCentre/HIVData/GlobalReport/Default.asp#english

UNDP (2000) *South Africa: Human Development Report* UNDP

USAID (2005) *Fragile States Strategy*. USAID: Washington

Whiteside, A. & Sunter, C. (2000) *AIDS: The challenge for South Africa*. Human & Rousseau: Johannesburg

World Bank (1999) *Local Government Responses to HIV/AIDS*. World Bank: Washington

INTERVIEWS

Hendrickse, Michael. Senior manager Electoral Democracy, Training and Legal Services, Independent Electoral Commission of South Africa, Pretoria. Interviewed 2008/05/26.

Maujane, Benjy. Project coordinator, Local Government Centre, Idasa. Interviewed 2008/05/19.

LEGISLATION

Local Government Transition Act (No. 209 of 1993)
Municipal Structures Act (No. 117 of 1998)
Municipal Systems Act (No. 32 of 2000)
Public Funding of Represented Political Parties Act (No. 103 of 1997)
The South African Constitution (1996)

NEWSPAPER ARTICLES

Mail & Guardian 2008/06/26: 'Local government spending black hole', Rossow, M.
The Star 2008/05/20: 'Budget will force power, water rethink', Cox, A.
The Star 2008/05/21: 'Lack of delivery partly to blame for the violence', Rabinowitz, R.
Sunday Times 2008/09/21: 'Wealthy restrict AIDS researchers', Keaton, C.

CONFERENCES

South-Eastern Europe Ministerial Conference (2004) 'Effective Democratic Governance at the Local and Regional Level'. Zagreb, Croatia. 25-26 October.

APPENDIX

KwaZulu-Natal matrix

Institutional response to HIV/AIDS			
	Bergville Okhahlamba Local Municipality	Ladysmith Emnambithi-Ladysmith Local Municipality	Richards Bay uMhlathuze Local Municipality
Workplace policy	6/10 yes 2/10 no 1/10 unsure 1/10 no answer *We definitely do need a freestanding HIV policy.*	11/14 yes 1/14 no 1/14 unsure 1/14 no answer 11/18 yes 1/18 no 3/18 unsure 3/18 no answer	
When policy was implemented	Information not provided.	Information not provided.	Information not provided.
Defined role of councillor under all respondents	In terms of legislation 5/10 yes 4/10 no 1/10 not applicable	9/14 yes 2/14 no 3/14 unsure	5/14 yes 6/14 no 3/14 unsure *There is no defined role, actually we are just working …*
Clinics	Available with VCT, ARVs and PMTCT for pregnant mothers. *Our clinics provide ARVs to the community.*	Available with services and programmes that deal with HIV/AIDS; they educate people and introduce ARVs.	Available with testing centres and free condoms; opened once a week; ARVs are also provided. *At all our clinics, ARVs are being supplied.*
Medical aid schemes	5/10 yes 4/10 no 1/10 not applicable *Not all staff; those who are on medical aid can afford it but there are people who are below the breadline who can't afford medical aid.*	7/15 yes, private 4/15 yes municipality 4/15 no *There is a medical aid scheme for officials or employees. I am not quite sure about councillors. They do get an allowance for themselves to get either their own scheme for medical aid or other benefits.*	7/15 yes, private 7/15 yes, municipality 0/15 no *I used to be a member of Bonitas but then I stopped the medical aid because it exploited me so much. I do not like medical aids any more.*

Anti-retroviral programmes	Available. *Provided at provincial hospitals and collected on a monthly basis.*	Available in clinics and Riebeeck Hospital. *There are not many people who take treatment here. Most people die because they do not want to disclose. I don't trust the ARVs as people are dying. We still rely on traditional help to help the people.*	Available to individuals with a CD4 count below 200. Have to travel to Welkom to get them.
Home-based care programmes	By trained volunteers. *It is not our issue to go to see people who are infected and affected, but in our meetings, we highlight the issue of HIV/AIDS.*	Available in conjunction with the Department of Health. It involves health workers, volunteers and support groups. *It is an unfunded mandate by the government.*	Conducted by NGOs, but assisted by the municipality. Churches and sisters at the clinics are also involved.
Orphans	Assisted through food parcels and tuition fees. *Our municipality is giving out food parcels to orphans. We have given another woman now money to gather those children and put them in a home and take care of them. It is non-governmental organisations, it is NGOs and MPO, they provide another wing which supplies orphans with school uniforms, fees, fruits, veggies, and take the kids out for a ride, trips to the mountains, heritage sites.*	Assisted, in conjunction with social development, through food vouchers, blankets. There is also an orphanage. They have to fill out forms to obtain help from the municipality.	Assisted. Due to the lack of funds, RDP houses are built for them. Some are orphaned at Shilem and others continue in child-headed households. However, they do not pay rates and are given free electricity. *We assist the orphans in different ways.*

Impact on political and administrative systems			
	Bergville Okhahlamba Local Municipality	Ladysmith Emnambithi-Ladysmith Local Municipality	Richards Bay uMhlathuze Local Municipality
Loss of staff/ councillors	1 councillor lost to natural causes; 2 resigned. *I've lost a number of staff. If the person dies, it becomes hard to tell whether it was HIV/AIDS related, but we have lost a couple of lives to illnesses that were uncertain.*	*You have people that have actually passed on and have to be replaced by new people.*	2 councillors lost. *Councillors are sick and are really dying. We lose a lot of staff members. We have lost people to AIDS because the infection rate has increased and that also applies to our workforce. We have lost people with skills and experience There have been deaths within the municipality, staff leaving. I have lost a colleague, but I don't want to mention his name.*
Absenteeism	Very high. *But in the meantime, they are absent and there is a void at the workplace; it definitely affects the workplace.*	Very high. *Once people are sick, you know that they cannot perform in terms of productivity levels that are expected of them. They are not getting anywhere too, but you cannot get them out of the system and, as a result, productivity levels are extremely low.*	Very high. *It also impacts on productivity, because some people get sick and cannot work. They are off frequently from work. HIV affects one of our members and they are sick and not able to continue with work.*
Service delivery	Affected by the lack of capacity, few or a lack of staff. Problems are in terms of the broader network and inadequate infrastructure. *So it affects us negatively.*	The municipality's performance and production levels are affected by absenteeism, loss of staff, lack of employment and poor infrastructure.	Affected by productivity issues, absenteeism, lack of education, unemployment, and proper roads, water and sanitation, crime, housing, the elderly, unemployment and poverty.
Development of sustainable programmes	Awareness through meetings, road shows and workshops. *There are good programmes and we have also increased about 30% for this financial year's budget, so that there are programmes pertaining to HIV/AIDS.*	Through workshops in Collinsville, municipal employee counselling, VCT, poverty alleviation project in the municipality, EAPs and awareness campaigns.	Establishment of the community safety forum, the AIDS Council in partnership with UNDP, and campaigns launched in association with the sisters at the clinic. Campaigns in Eshowe, distribution of food and medication, HIV/AIDS portfolio committee.

FREE STATE MATRIX

Institutional response to HIV/AIDS				
	Welkom Matjhabeng Local Municipality	Theunissen Masilonyana Local Municipality	Ladybrand Mantsopa Local Municipality	Clocolan/Ficksburg Setsoto Local Municipality
Workplace policy	2/23 do not know 21/23 yes	8/9 yes 1/9 no	7/9 yes 1/9 no 1/9 does not know	11/13 yes 2/13 do not know
When policy implemented	Information not provided.	Information not provided.	Information not provided.	Information not provided.
Defined role of councillor	17/23 yes 4/23 no 2/23 not questioned	6/9 yes 3/9 no *Completely no, there are no defined roles.*	5/9 yes 2/9 no 1/9 unsure 1/9 does not know	5/13 yes 4/13 no 2/13 unsure 1/13 does not know 1/13 no response
Clinics	Available. *Clinics are developing in my ward.*	Available. *They have no privacy. Everyone in the clinics will know your business. There is a lack of trust among clinic staff.*	Available, with free condoms.	Available, with ARVs and counselling. *We have a clinic, but it refers people to a clinic in Marquard for treatment.*
Medical aid schemes	5/23 no 18/23 yes *Medical aid is for all the members of the municipality.*	5/9 yes (3 private) 4/9 no	6/9 yes 2/9 no 1/9 no response	10/13 yes (4 private) 1/13 no 2/13 no response
Anti-retroviral programmes	Available and distributed to the needy, and follow-ups are done to monitor them. *ARVs, it is helping, but it takes long for the clinics to get it to those people. Some die before they can get it.*	Available in Welkom and Bloemfontein. *People from our municipality don't have to travel out of the municipality ... to get hold of this medication, so that it can be dished out.*	*We have an ARV centre here in Ladybrand.*	New centre opened up. *We have an ARV centre. If they are diagnosed, there at the clinic, they go for ARVs.*
Home-based care programmes	Volunteers go from door to door. They also assist with the taking of medication.	Through the help of volunteers, provincial government, employees from the Department of Health, and a woman's organisation of 12 people. *Volunteers give people the treatment at their homes.*	*Yes we do have home-based care, almost all of us.*	SAPO. In collaboration with the Department of Health who have caregivers and nurses. *There is a lot of work that has been done about home-based care.*

Orphans	Assisted. *There are orphans as a result of HIV/AIDS, whom I have adopted and help them to go to school, to buy uniforms and to see to it that they are getting food at the end of the day.*	There is a facility in Bramford. Department of Social Welfare helps find homes and register for grants. Community development worker – Khelo Sova. *... taking care of them, educating them, primary health care ...*	Receive grants, work with Managwe, MEC and the police. *Children head households because most of the parents have passed away because of this disease.*	There is a large number due to HIV/AIDS. Many child-headed households. *It leaves children as orphans. Children have to run the household and some end up as street children. Yes, we have a lot of children who have lost their parents as a result of HIV/AIDS.*

Impact on political and administrative systems				
	Welkom Matjhabeng Local Municipality	Theunissen Masilonyana Local Municipality	Ladybrand Mantsopa Local Municipality	Clocolan/Ficksburg Setsoto Local Municipality
Loss of staff/ councillors	*The staff is clearly demoralised because, sometimes, one of our popular councillors will get sick and die of it, and it affects the staff too much.*	*One died because she was sick. We are losing a number of employees to illness.*	A councillor resigned. *A few people have passed away, but not because of AIDS. Some of the symptoms are the same, but we don't know, because people don't disclose.*	*People are dying; you hear that they died of TB. Many stories, but we know its HIV. Yes we are losing staff really more especially in the technical department.*
Absenteeism	High. *Many people are kind of laid off because they are not feeling too well, so that affects even the economy of the municipality, but I must say, it will affect it in a great way, big way.*	High. *You get absenteeism, people who can't come to work because they are sick, suffering from pneumonia, suffering from TB, suffering from meningitis, stiffness in the neck. So many people don't come to work.*	High. *Now if I look here in our municipality, they getting infected, many people are not at work.*	High. *Many people at work have been put off for sick leave. Most people have been given leave because if someone is sick, they can't perform.*

Service delivery	Affected by developmental challenges, unemployment, sanitation, poverty. *We are having a sick society which is down because of HIV/AIDS. It means that we are going to have a little people paying our services, therefore we are going to be unable to render services as we are supposed to.*	Affected by developmental challenges such as crime, water and sanitation, child-headed households, poverty, HIV/AIDS. *So it does hamper service delivery in a sense.* *It is actually the fact that normal running is not there because of people who are sick.*	Affected by developmental challenges, unemployment, and sanitation. *The more people are sick, the more the municipality gets into problems, because people don't work and can't pay for services.*	Affected by developmental challenges such as education, unemployment, housing, HIV/AIDS, poverty. *It has a great impact because, when people are not working, they cannot pay for their services, so the municipality is making a loss.* *The people who are key people are the ones who are ill.*
Development of sustainable programmes	Workshops, assistance from NGOs, local AIDS council, AIDS forum.	Workshops, local AIDS council, NGOs – Mekele-kela Counter-AIDS Campaign, Love Life, community outreach programmes.	Local AIDS council, Manjupa forum.	AIDS budget awareness campaigns, HIV workshops in schools.

WESTERN CAPE MATRIX

Institutional response to HIV/AIDS		
	Piketberg Bergriver Local Municipality	Saldanha Bay Saldanha Bay Local Municipality
Workplace policy	1/3 yes 1/3 not questioned 1/3 does not know	4/5 yes 1/5 no
When policy implemented	Information not provided.	Information not provided.
Defined role of councillor	1/3 yes 1/3 not questioned 1/3 no	3/5 yes 1/5 no 1/5 not sure
Clinics	Available with VCT and TB medication.	Available with VCT centres and free condoms. *Six major towns in our municipality area and a clinic in each.*
Medical aid schemes	1/3 yes (private) 1/3 no 1/3 not questioned	All have medical aid.
Anti-retroviral programmes	Information not provided.	At clinics. *They all provide ARV treatment.*
Home-based care programmes	BMW programme provides food parcels, cleans houses and a clean environment.	Involves health caregivers who do the washing, and social workers who report any problems.
Orphans	Information not provided.	*I do not get requests for care and orphans support, not to my knowledge.*

Impact on political and administrative systems		
	Piketberg Bergriver Local Municipality	Saldanha Bay Saldanha Bay Local Municipality
Loss of staff/ councillors	Information not provided.	Loss due to death that was HIV/AIDS-related. *Yes, political leaders I know but I cannot disclose, it is confidential.*
Absenteeism	Information not provided.	High. *And when it comes to absenteeism, you do not know if it is AIDS-related or not.*
Service delivery	Lack of proper infrastructure, employment and investment has a negative impact on service delivery.	Affected by the backlog in infrastructure, drugs, alcoholism, education, low and lack of skills. *Municipality is a service tool, not a delivery tool. As a councillor, the national and provincial government must deliver.*
Development of sustainable programmes	BMW programme deals with home-based care.	Awareness programmes such as Love Life, workshops with NGOs, HIV/AIDS support group.

NORTHERN CAPE MATRIX

Institutional response to HIV/AIDS			
	Kimberley Sol Plaatjie Local Municipality	Warrenton Magareng Local Municipality	Springbok/Steinkopf Nama Khoi Local Municipality
Workplace policy	9/10 yes 1/10 unsure A copy of the policy was given.	2/5 yes 2/5 no 1/5 unaware *Within the ANC I believe there must be, within the municipality, we must have a draft.*	8/9 yes 1/9 no
When policy implemented	Information not provided.	Information not provided.	Information not provided.
Defined role of councillor	4/9 yes 3/9 no 1/9 not sure 1/9 unaware	3/5 no 1/5 unsure 1/5 no response *No role, just responsibility to encourage awareness and lead by example.*	2/9 yes 7/9 no *There isn't a role as a community leader.*
Clinics	Available. *Clinics are hopelessly inadequate.*	Available, with VCT centre and free condoms.	Available, with Santa-TB and food parcels. *The clinics and hospitals are doing their best to treat these people.*
Medical aid schemes	9/10 yes 1/10 no	3/5 yes 1/5 no 1/5 no response 60% subsidy and 40% contribution.	4/9 yes (private) 4/9 no 1/9 not questioned *At this point, medical aid is voluntary and there is a system for those who do not have a medical aid.*
Anti-retroviral programmes	Distributed only to individuals with a CD4 count below 200. *Clinics are certainly inadequate with this problem. On a small scale.* *They are given to employee and his/her partner.*	Distributed at the hospital. *Some clinics do not have and people have to travel to Kimberley.*	Available. *The treatment is not what it should be.*
Home-based care programmes	Rotary Club, William Humphrey Art Gallery training, soup kitchen and daily feeding scheme.	CBO home-based centre, Boitumelo, conducted by support groups and NGOs.	Conducted by volunteers, home caregivers who feed people, clean their houses and support families. R1 000 grant per month. *Homecare givers are to ensure that the drugs are taken and that there are people to provide care.*